# MEATLESS

**DELICIOUS RECIPES FOR EVERY MEAL**

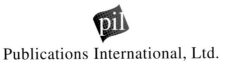

Publications International, Ltd.

**Pictured on the front cover:** Peanut Butter Tofu Bowl *(page 106)*.

**Pictured on the back cover** *(clockwise from top right):* Double Decker Tacos *(page 62)*, Vegetarian Lasagna *(page 98)*, Minestrone Soup *(page 158)* and Roasted Brussels Sprouts Salad *(page 29)*.

ISBN: 978-1-64558-252-6

Manufactured in China.

8 7 6 5 4 3 2 1

**Let's get social!**
🄾 @Publications_International
🄵 @PublicationsInternational
**www.pilbooks.com**

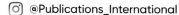

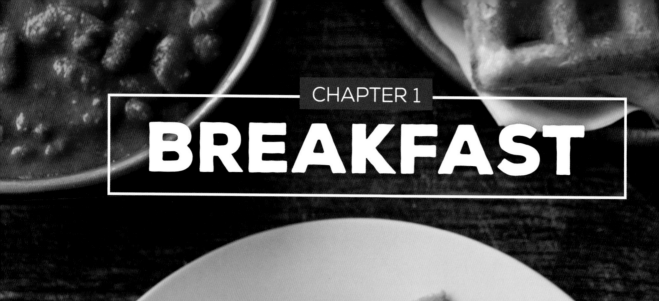

# CHAPTER 1

# BREAKFAST

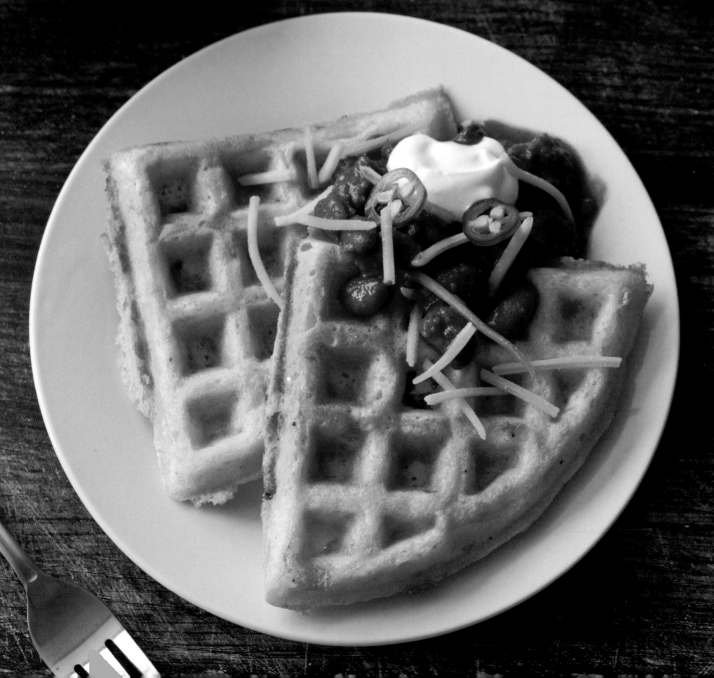

# CHEDDAR JALAPEÑO CORNMEAL WAFFLES

1¼ cups yellow cornmeal

¾ cup all-purpose flour

2 tablespoons sugar

2 teaspoons baking powder

1 teaspoon salt

½ teaspoon baking soda

¾ cup (3 ounces) shredded sharp Cheddar cheese

1 jalapeño pepper, sliced into thin rings

2 eggs

2 cups buttermilk

6 tablespoons butter, melted and slightly cooled

**1.** Preheat oven to 200°F. Preheat classic waffle maker to medium-high heat. Set wire rack on large baking sheet.

**2.** Whisk cornmeal, flour, sugar, baking powder, salt and baking soda in large bowl until combined. Fold in cheese and jalapeño pepper.

**3.** Whisk eggs in medium bowl. Add buttermilk and butter, whisk until well blended. Pour buttermilk mixture into flour mixture; stir until combined.

**4.** Pour ½ cup batter into center of waffle maker; close lid and cook about 3 to 5 minutes or until golden brown and crisp. Remove to wire rack; keep warm in oven. Repeat with remaining batter.

**MAKES 8 SERVINGS**

TIP

Serve with a bowl of chili. Or, reheat leftovers and serve with salsa and avocado.

# SWEET POTATO PANCAKES

## PANCAKES

- **2 medium sweet potatoes**
- **2½ cups all-purpose flour**
- **1 teaspoon baking powder**
- **1 teaspoon baking soda**
- **½ teaspoon salt**
- **½ teaspoon ground cinnamon**
- **¼ teaspoon ground ginger**
- **2¾ cups buttermilk**
- **2 eggs**
- **2 tablespoons packed brown sugar**
- **2 tablespoons butter, melted, plus additional for pan**

## GINGER BUTTER

- **¼ cup (½ stick) butter, softened**
- **1 tablespoon packed brown sugar**
- **1 teaspoon grated fresh ginger**
- **Pinch salt**
- **Prepared caramel sauce or maple syrup**
- **¾ cup chopped glazed pecans***

*\*Glazed or candied pecans can be found in the produce section of the supermarket with other salad toppings, or they may be in the snack aisle.*

**1.** Preheat oven to 375°F. Scrub sweet potatoes; bake 50 to 60 minutes or until soft. Cool slightly; peel and mash. Measure 1⅓ cups for pancake batter.

**2.** Combine flour, baking powder, baking soda, salt, cinnamon and ground ginger in medium bowl; mix well. Whisk buttermilk, eggs and 2 tablespoons brown sugar in large bowl until well blended. Stir in melted butter. Add sweet potato; whisk until well blended. Add flour mixture; stir just until dry ingredients are moistened and no streaks of flour remain. Do not overmix; batter will be lumpy. Let stand 10 minutes.

**3.** Heat griddle or large skillet* over medium heat; brush with additional melted butter to coat. For each pancake, pour ½ cup of batter onto griddle, spreading into 5- to 6-inch circle. Cook about 4 minutes or until bottom is golden brown and small bubbles appear on surface. Turn pancake; cook about 3 minutes or until golden brown. Add additional butter to griddle as needed.

**4.** For ginger butter, beat ¼ cup softened butter, 1 tablespoon brown sugar, fresh ginger and pinch of salt in small bowl until well blended. If using caramel sauce, microwave according to package directions. Stir in water, 1 teaspoon at a time, to thin to desired pouring consistency.

**5.** Serve pancakes warm topped with glazed pecans, ginger butter and caramel sauce.

## MAKES 5 SERVINGS (10 LARGE PANCAKES)

*\*Since pancakes are large, a skillet may not be able to cook more than one at a time. Keep cooked pancakes warm in 250°F oven on wire rack set over baking sheet.*

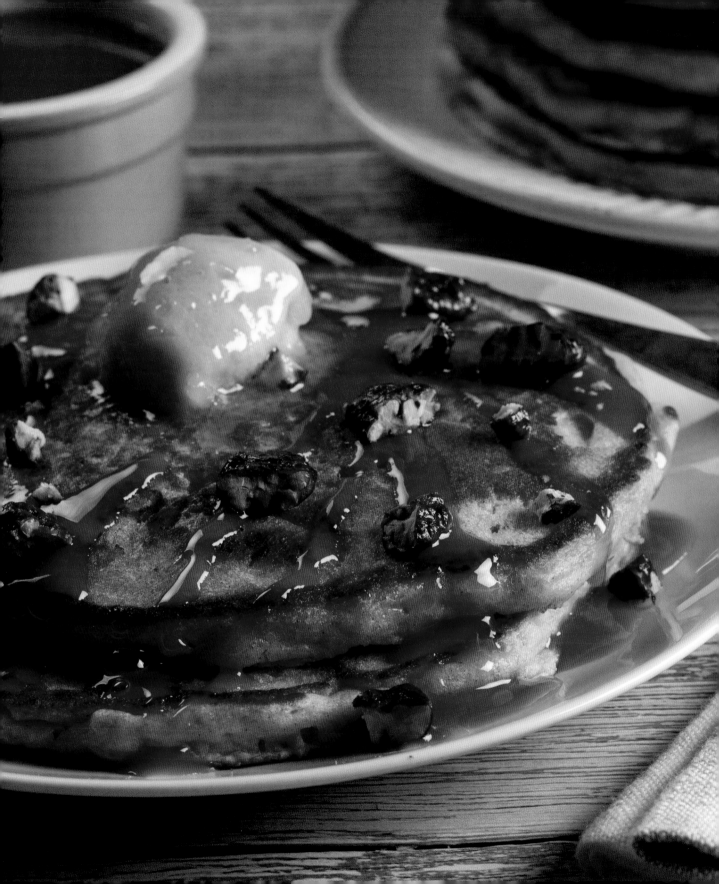

# CHEESY QUICHETTES

1 package (5¼ ounces) veggie bacon strips, cooked according to package directions and finely chopped

6 eggs, beaten

¼ cup whole milk

1½ cups thawed frozen shredded hash brown potatoes, squeezed dry

¼ cup chopped fresh parsley

½ teaspoon salt

1½ cups (6 ounces) shredded Mexican cheese blend with jalapeño peppers

**1.** Preheat oven to 400°F. Lightly spray 12 standard (2½-inch) muffin cups with nonstick cooking spray.

**2.** Divide bacon evenly among prepared muffin cups. Beat eggs and milk in medium bowl. Add potatoes, parsley and salt; mix well. Spoon mixture evenly into muffin cups.

**3.** Bake 15 minutes or until knife inserted into centers comes out almost clean. Sprinkle evenly with cheese; let stand 3 minutes or until cheese is melted. (Egg mixture will continue to cook while standing.) Gently run knife around edges and lift out with fork.

**MAKES 12 QUICHETTES**

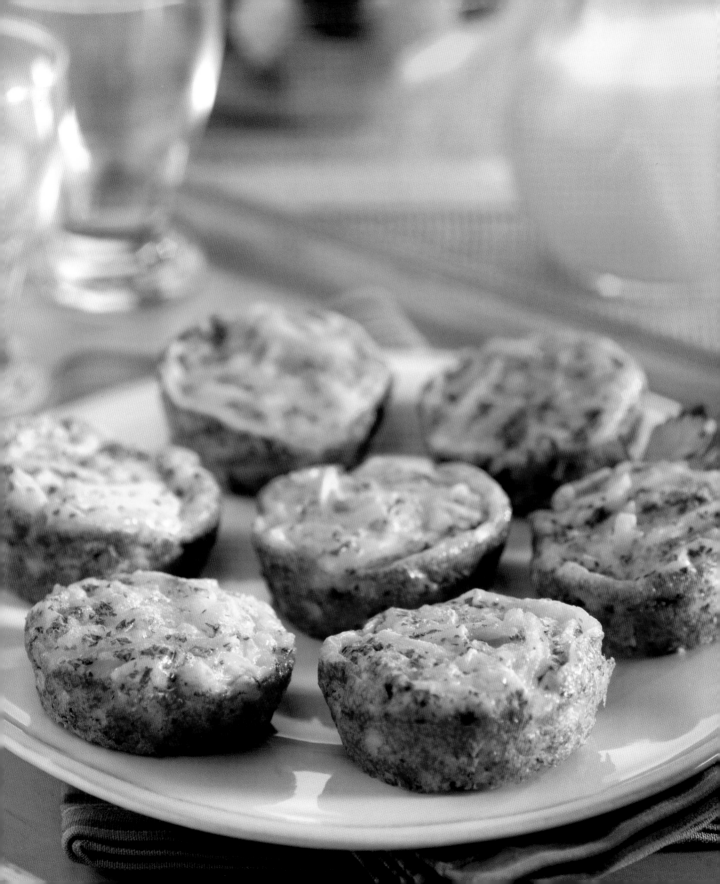

# BANANA-BLUEBERRY OAT AND QUINOA SNACK CAKE

- **2** cups old-fashioned oats
- **1** cup uncooked quinoa, rinsed well in fine-mesh strainer
- **1** cup packed dark brown sugar, divided
- **⅔** cup all-purpose flour
- **1½** teaspoons ground cinnamon
- **1½** teaspoons baking powder
- **½** teaspoon salt
- **3** medium ripe bananas
- **1** cup milk
- **2** eggs
- **½** cup applesauce
- **2** tablespoons butter, melted
- **½** teaspoon vanilla
- **2** cups fresh blueberries, divided
- **½** cup chopped pecans

**1.** Preheat oven to 375°F. Spray 13×9-inch baking pan with nonstick cooking spray.

**2.** Combine oats, quinoa, ¾ cup brown sugar, flour, cinnamon, baking powder and salt in large bowl.

**3.** Mash bananas in medium bowl. Stir in milk, eggs, applesauce, butter and vanilla. Add to quinoa mixture; mix well. Fold in 1 cup blueberries. Spread batter in prepared pan; sprinkle with remaining blueberries, remaining ¼ cup brown sugar and pecans.

**4.** Bake 40 to 45 minutes or until golden brown and set. Cool in pan 10 minutes before serving. Serve warm or at room temperature. Store leftovers in refrigerator.

**MAKES 8 SERVINGS**

**TIP**

Vegan Swaps: Oat milk for regular milk, vegan plant butter for regular butter and flax for eggs (combine 2 tablespoons ground flaxseed and 6 tablespoons boiling water in small bowl; cool completely before using).

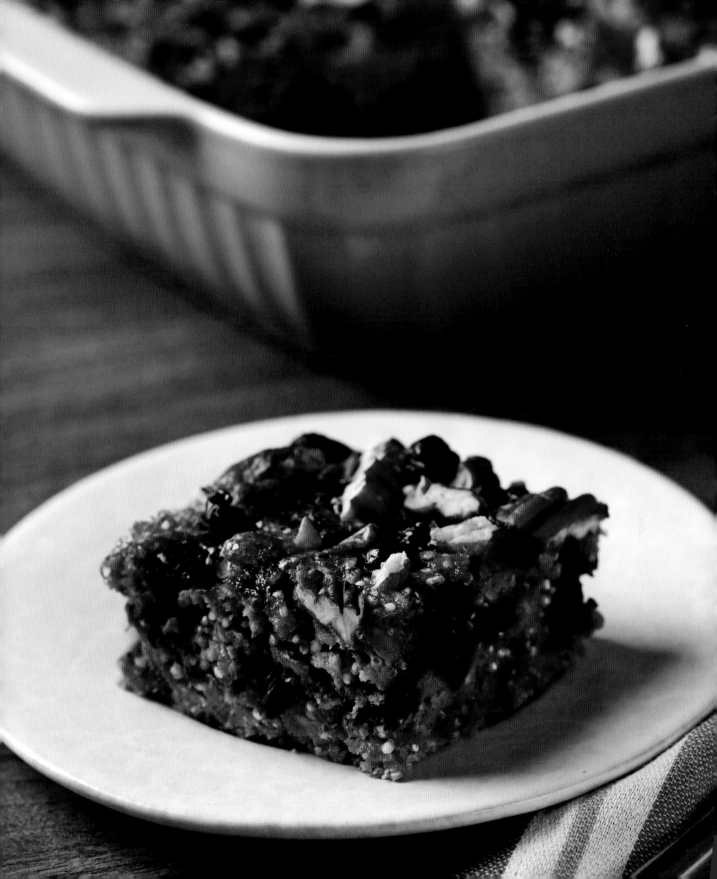

# STRAWBERRY-TOPPED PANCAKES

1½ **cups sliced fresh strawberries**

2 **tablespoons seedless strawberry jam**

1¼ **cups all-purpose flour**

¼ **cup sugar**

1 **teaspoon baking powder**

1 **teaspoon baking soda**

¼ **teaspoon salt**

1¼ **cups buttermilk**

1 **egg**

1 **to 2 tablespoons vegetable oil**

**Whipped cream (optional)**

**1.** Combine strawberries and strawberry jam in medium bowl; stir gently to coat. Set aside while preparing pancakes.

**2.** Combine flour, sugar, baking powder, baking soda and salt in large bowl; mix well. Add buttermilk and egg; whisk until blended.

**3.** Heat 1 tablespoon oil in large skillet over medium heat or brush griddle with oil. For each pancake, pour ½ cup of batter into skillet, spreading into 5- to 6-inch circle. Cook 3 to 4 minutes or until bottom is golden brown and small bubbles appear on surface. Turn pancake; cook 2 minutes or until golden brown. Add additional oil to skillet as needed.

**4.** For each serving, stack three pancakes; top with strawberry mixture. Garnish with whipped cream.

**MAKES 2 SERVINGS (6 LARGE PANCAKES)**

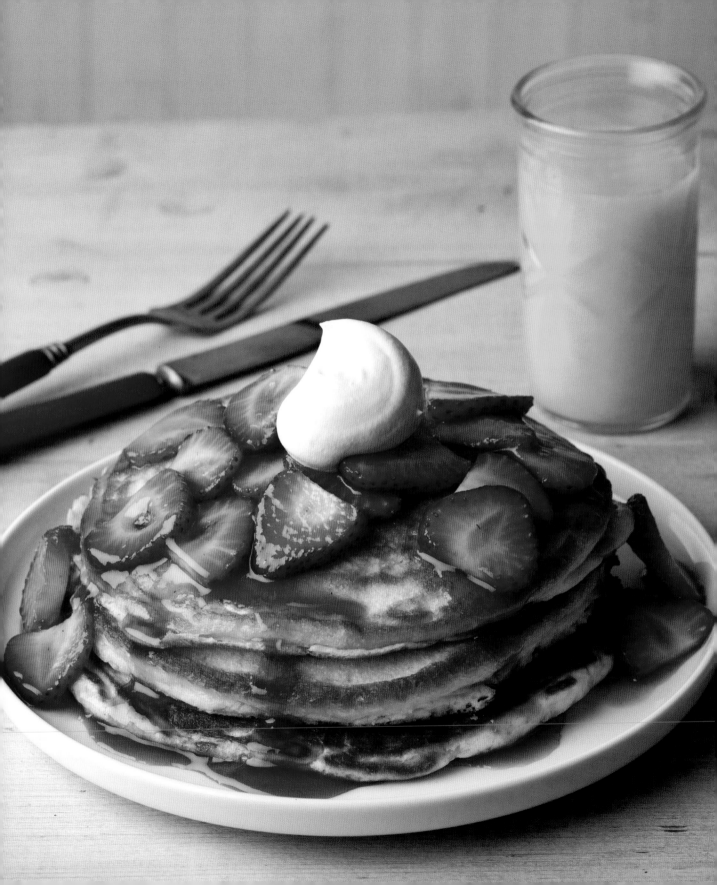

# FRITTATA RUSTICA

- **4** ounces cremini mushrooms, stems trimmed, cut into thirds
- **1** tablespoon olive oil, divided
- **½** teaspoon plus ⅛ teaspoon salt, divided
- **½** cup chopped onion
- **1** cup packed chopped stemmed lacinato kale
- **½** cup halved grape tomatoes
- **4** eggs
- **½** teaspoon Italian seasoning
- Black pepper
- **⅓** cup shredded mozzarella cheese
- **1** tablespoon shredded Parmesan cheese
- Chopped fresh parsley

**1.** Preheat oven to 400°F. Spread mushrooms on small baking sheet; drizzle with 1 teaspoon oil and sprinkle with ⅛ teaspoon salt. Roast 15 to 20 minutes or until well browned and tender.

**2.** Heat remaining 2 teaspoons oil in small (6- to 8-inch) nonstick skillet over medium heat. Add onion; cook and stir 5 minutes or until soft. Add kale and ¼ teaspoon salt; cook and stir 10 minutes or until kale is tender. Add tomatoes; cook and stir 3 minutes or until tomatoes are soft. Stir in mushrooms.

**3.** Preheat broiler. Whisk eggs, remaining ¼ teaspoon salt, Italian seasoning and pepper in small bowl until well blended.

**4.** Pour egg mixture over vegetables in skillet; stir gently to mix. Cook about 3 minutes or until eggs are set around edge, lifting edge to allow uncooked portion to flow underneath. Sprinkle with mozzarella and Parmesan. Broil 3 minutes or until eggs are set and cheese is browned. Sprinkle with parsley.

**MAKES 2 SERVINGS**

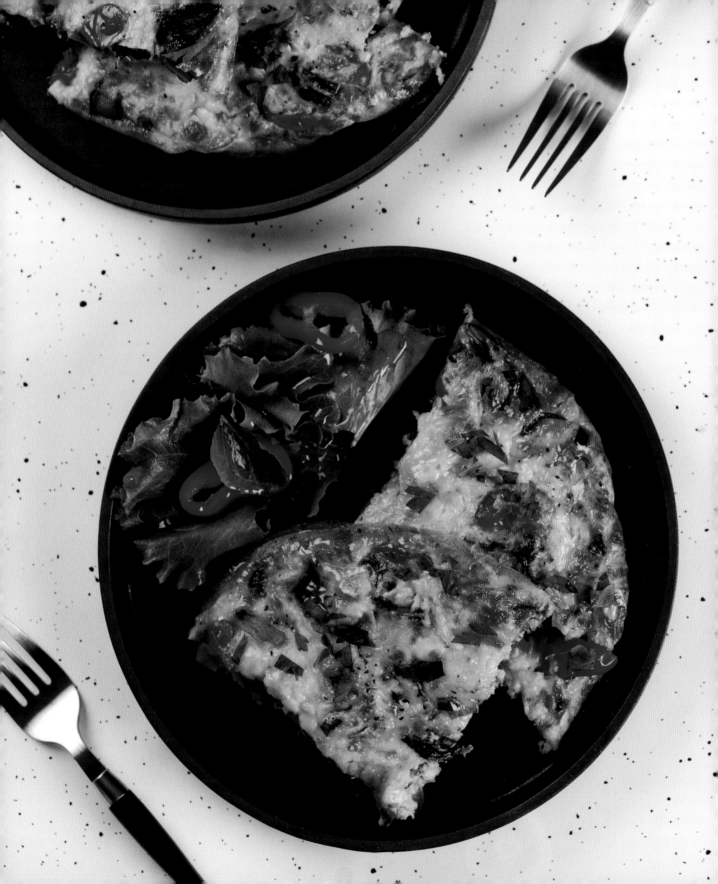

# BAKED APPLE PANCAKE

3 tablespoons butter

3 medium Granny Smith apples (about 1¼ pounds), peeled and cut into ¼-inch slices

½ cup packed dark brown sugar

1½ teaspoons ground cinnamon

½ teaspoon plus pinch of salt, divided

4 eggs

⅓ cup whipping cream

⅓ cup milk

2 tablespoons granulated sugar

½ teaspoon vanilla

⅔ cup all-purpose flour

**1.** Melt butter in 8-inch ovenproof nonstick or cast iron skillet over medium heat. Add apples, brown sugar, cinnamon and pinch of salt; cook about 8 minutes or until apples begin to soften, stirring occasionally. Spread apples in even layer in skillet; set aside to cool 30 minutes.

**2.** After apples have cooled 30 minutes, preheat oven to 425°F. Whisk eggs in large bowl until foamy. Add cream, milk, granulated sugar, vanilla and remaining ½ teaspoon salt; whisk until blended. Sift flour into egg mixture; whisk until batter is well blended and smooth. Set aside 15 minutes.

**3.** Stir batter; pour evenly over apple mixture. Place skillet on rimmed baking sheet in case of drips (or place baking sheet or piece of foil in oven beneath skillet).

**4.** Bake about 16 minutes or until top is golden brown and pancake is loose around edge. Cool 1 minute; loosen edge of pancake with spatula, if necessary. Place large serving plate or cutting board on top of skillet and invert pancake onto plate. Serve warm.

**MAKES 2 TO 4 SERVINGS**

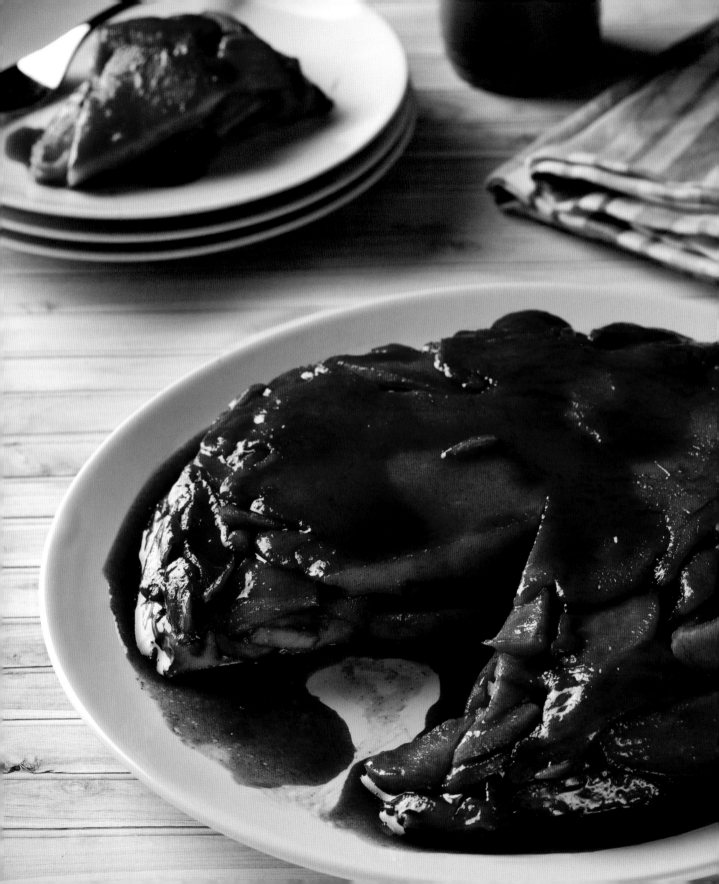

# STRAWBERRY BANANA FRENCH TOAST

1 cup sliced fresh
   strawberries
   (about 8 medium)

2 teaspoons granulated
   sugar

2 eggs

½ cup milk

3 tablespoons all-
   purpose flour

1 teaspoon vanilla

⅛ teaspoon salt

1 tablespoon butter,
   divided

4 slices (1 inch thick) egg
   bread or country
   bread

1 banana, cut into ¼-inch
   slices

   Whipped cream and
   powdered sugar
   (optional)

   Maple syrup

**1.** Combine strawberries and granulated sugar in small bowl; toss to coat. Set aside while preparing French toast.

**2.** Whisk eggs, milk, flour, vanilla and salt in shallow bowl or pie plate until well blended. Melt ½ tablespoon butter in large skillet over medium-high heat. Working with 2 slices at a time, dip bread into egg mixture, turning to coat completely; let excess drip off. Add to skillet; cook 3 to 4 minutes per side or until golden brown. Repeat with remaining butter and bread slices.

**3.** Top each serving with strawberry mixture and banana slices. Garnish with whipped cream and powdered sugar; serve with maple syrup.

**MAKES 2 SERVINGS**

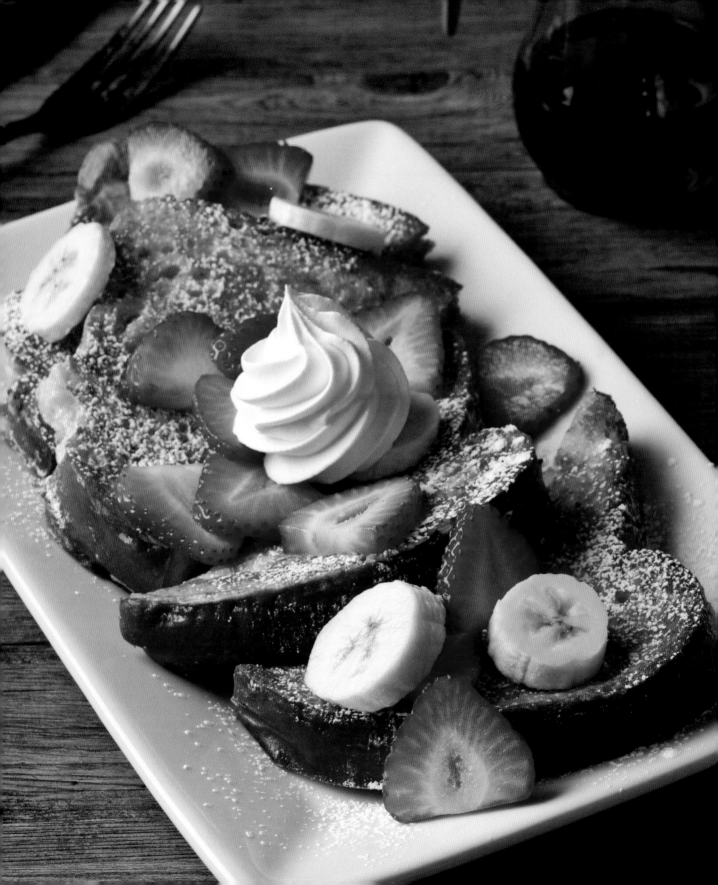

# PECAN WAFFLES

2¼ cups all-purpose flour

3 tablespoons sugar

1 tablespoon baking powder

½ teaspoon salt

2 cups milk

2 eggs, beaten

¼ cup vegetable oil

¾ cup chopped pecans, toasted*

Butter and maple syrup for serving

*To toast pecans, cook in medium skillet over medium heat 3 to 4 minutes or until lightly browned, stirring frequently.

**1.** Preheat classic round waffle iron; grease lightly.

**2.** Combine flour, sugar, baking powder and salt in large bowl. Whisk milk, eggs and oil in medium bowl until well blended. Add to flour mixture; stir just until blended. Stir in pecans.

**3.** For each waffle, pour about ½ cup batter into waffle iron. Close lid and bake until steaming stops. Serve with butter and maple syrup.

**MAKES 8 WAFFLES**

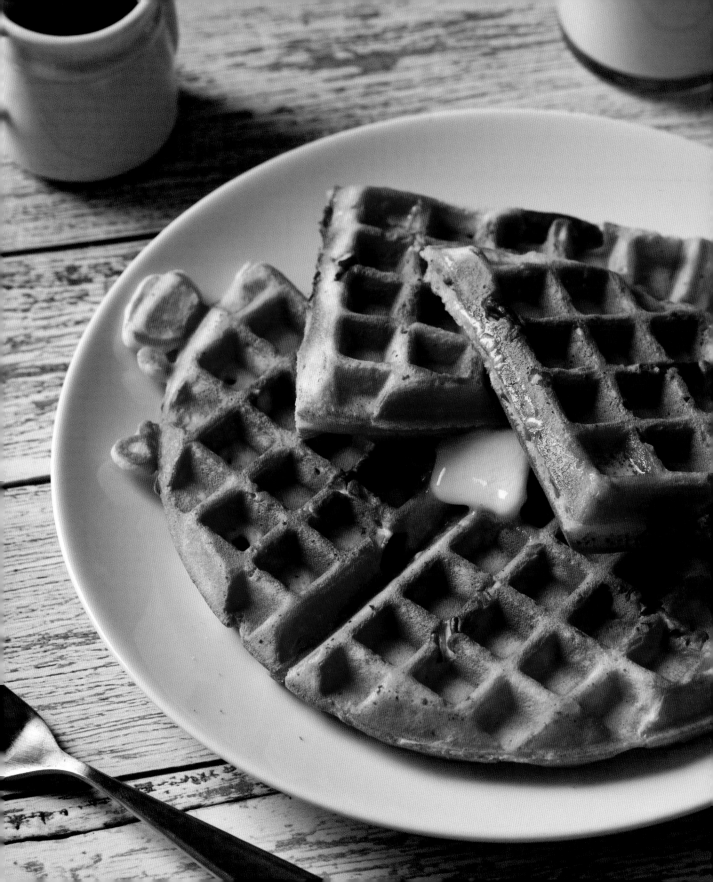

# FRENCH CARROT QUICHE

- **1 pound carrots**
- **1 tablespoon butter**
- **¼ cup chopped green onions**
- **½ teaspoon herbes de Provence**
- **1 cup milk**
- **¼ cup whipping cream**
- **½ cup all-purpose flour**
- **2 eggs, lightly beaten**
- **½ teaspoon minced fresh thyme**
- **¼ teaspoon ground nutmeg**
- **½ cup (2 ounces) shredded Gruyère or Swiss cheese**

**1.** Peel carrots and cut into rounds. Butter four shallow 1-cup baking dishes or one 9-inch quiche dish or shallow casserole. Preheat oven to 350°F.

**2.** Melt butter in large skillet over medium heat. Cook and stir carrots, green onions and herbes de Provence 3 to 4 minutes or until carrots are tender.

**3.** Meanwhile, combine milk and cream in medium bowl; whisk in flour gradually. Stir in eggs, thyme and nutmeg.

**4.** Spread carrot mixture in prepared dishes; add milk mixture. Sprinkle with cheese. Bake 20 to 25 minutes for individual quiches or 30 to 40 minutes for 9-inch quiche or until firm. Serve warm or at room temperature.

**MAKES 4 SERVINGS**

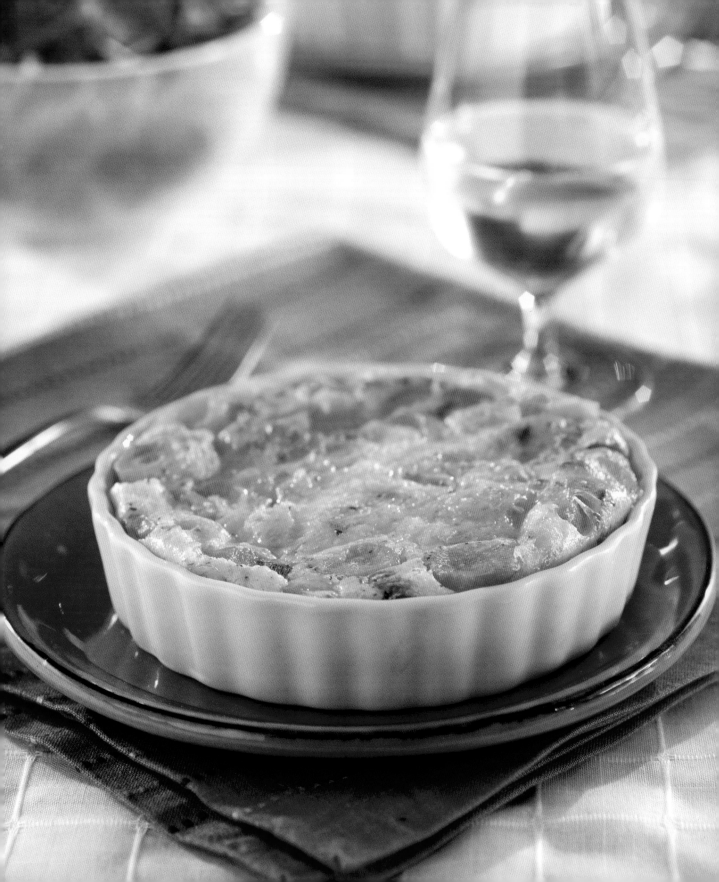

# CRANBERRY WALNUT GRANOLA BARS

2 cups old-fashioned oats

¾ cup all-purpose flour

1 teaspoon pumpkin pie spice

½ teaspoon baking soda

½ teaspoon salt

1 cup packed brown sugar

¼ cup (½ stick) butter, softened

2 eggs

¼ cup orange juice

1 cup chopped walnuts

½ cup dried cranberries

**1.** Preheat oven to 350°F. Spray 9-inch square baking pan with nonstick cooking spray.

**2.** Combine oats, flour, pumpkin pie spice, baking soda and salt in medium bowl.

**3.** Beat brown sugar and butter in large bowl with electric mixer on medium-high speed until light and fluffy. Add eggs and orange juice; beat until blended. Gradually add oat mixture, beating just until mixed. Stir in walnuts and cranberries. Spread mixture in prepared pan.

**4.** Bake 20 to 25 minutes or until toothpick inserted into center comes out clean. Cool completely in pan. Cut into bars.

**MAKES 12 BARS**

**TIP**

Vegan Swaps: Vegan plant butter for regular butter and flax for eggs (combine 2 tablespoons ground flaxseed and 6 tablespoons boiling water in small bowl; cool completely before using).

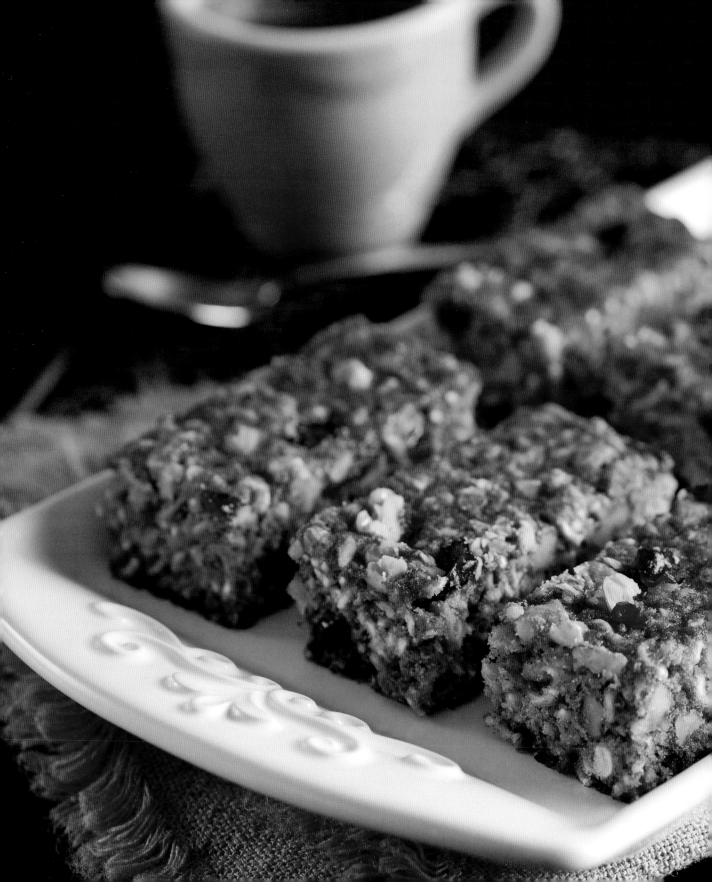

# AVOCADO TOAST

½ cup thawed frozen
   peas

2 teaspoons lemon juice

1 teaspoon minced fresh
   tarragon

¼ teaspoon plus
   ⅛ teaspoon salt,
   divided

⅛ teaspoon black pepper

1 teaspoon olive oil

1 tablespoon raw
   pepitas (pumpkin
   seeds)

4 slices hearty whole
   grain bread, toasted

1 avocado

**1.** Combine peas, lemon juice, tarragon, ¼ teaspoon salt and pepper in small food processor; pulse until blended but still chunky. Or combine all ingredients in small bowl and mash with fork to desired consistency.

**2.** Heat oil in small saucepan over medium heat. Add pepitas; cook and stir 1 to 2 minutes or until toasted. Transfer to small bowl; stir in remaining ⅛ teaspoon salt.

**3.** Spread about 1 tablespoon pea mixture over each slice of bread. If making one serving, place the remaining pea mixture in a jar or container and store in the refrigerator for a day or two.

**4.** Cut avocado in half lengthwise around pit. If making one serving, wrap the half with the pit in plastic wrap and store in the refrigerator for a day or two. Cut the avocado into slices in the shell; use a spoon to scoop the slices out of the shell. Arrange the slices on the toast; top with toasted pepitas.

**MAKES 2 SERVINGS**

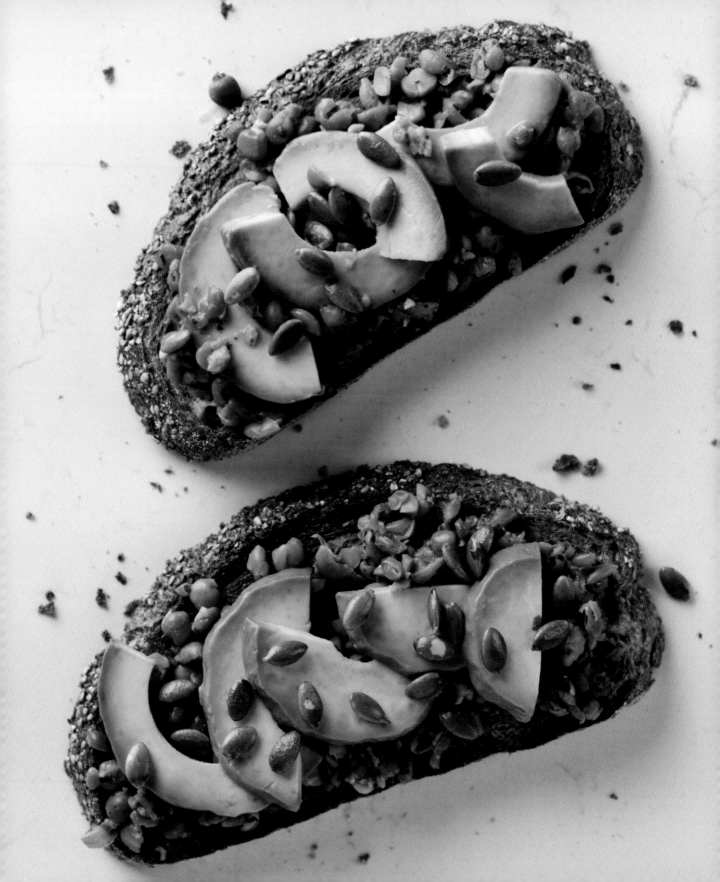

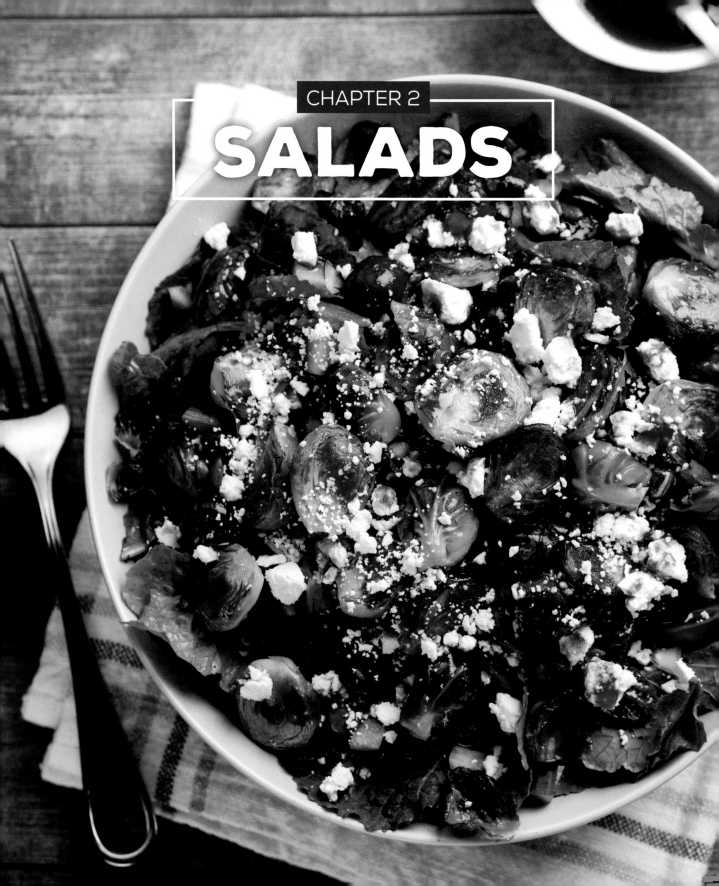

# CHAPTER 2

# SALADS

# ROASTED BRUSSELS SPROUTS SALAD

## BRUSSELS SPROUTS

- 1 pound brussels sprouts, trimmed and halved
- 2 tablespoons olive oil
- ½ teaspoon salt

## SALAD

- 2 cups coarsely chopped baby kale
- 2 cups coarsely chopped romaine lettuce
- 1½ cups candied pecans*
- 1 cup halved red grapes
- 1 cup diced cucumbers
- ½ cup dried cranberries
- ½ cup fresh blueberries
- ½ cup chopped red onion
- ¼ cup toasted pepitas (pumpkin seeds)
- 4 ounces crumbled goat cheese

## DRESSING

- ½ cup olive oil
- 6 tablespoons balsamic vinegar
- 6 tablespoons strawberry jam
- 2 teaspoons Dijon mustard
- 1 teaspoon salt

*Candied or glazed pecans can be found in the produce section of many supermarkets (with other salad toppings). If unavailable, they can easily be made at home. (See Tip on page 34.)

**1.** For brussels sprouts, preheat oven to 400°F. Spray large baking sheet with nonstick cooking spray.

**2.** Combine brussels sprouts, 2 tablespoons oil and ½ teaspoon salt in medium bowl; toss to coat. Arrange brussels sprouts in single layer, cut sides down, on prepared baking sheet. Roast 20 minutes or until tender and browned, stirring once halfway through roasting. Cool completely on baking sheet.

**3.** For salad, combine kale, lettuce, pecans, grapes, cucumbers, cranberries, blueberries, red onion and pepitas in large bowl. Top with brussels sprouts and cheese.

**4.** For dressing, whisk ½ cup oil, vinegar, jam, mustard and 1 teaspoon salt in small bowl until well blended. Pour over salad; toss gently to blend.

### MAKES 6 SERVINGS (ABOUT 8 CUPS)

**TIP**

Vegan Swaps: Omit the goat cheese or replace it with coarsely chopped toasted cashews or cubed smoked tofu.

# STEAKHOUSE CHOPPED SALAD

## DRESSING*

- 1½ teaspoons salt
- 1½ teaspoons dried oregano
- ¾ teaspoon sugar
- ¾ teaspoon onion powder
- ¾ teaspoon dried parsley flakes
- ½ teaspoon garlic powder
- ¼ teaspoon dried basil
- ¼ teaspoon black pepper
- ⅛ teaspoon dried thyme
- ⅛ teaspoon celery salt
- ⅓ cup white balsamic vinegar
- ¼ cup Dijon mustard
- ⅔ cup extra virgin olive oil

## SALAD

- 1 medium head iceberg lettuce, chopped
- 1 medium head romaine lettuce, chopped
- 1 can (about 14 ounces) hearts of palm or artichoke hearts, quartered lengthwise then sliced crosswise
- 1 large avocado, diced
- 1½ cups crumbled blue cheese
- 2 hard-cooked eggs, chopped
- 1 ripe tomato, chopped
- ½ small red onion, finely chopped
- 1 package (5¼ ounces) veggie bacon strips, cooked according to package directions and chopped

*Or substitute 1 package (about 2 tablespoons) Italian salad dressing mix for the seasonings in the dressing.

**1.** For dressing, combine salt, oregano, sugar, onion powder, parsley flakes, garlic powder, basil, pepper, thyme and celery salt in medium bowl. Whisk in vinegar and mustard. Slowly add oil, whisking until well blended. Set aside until ready to use. (Dressing can be made up to 1 week in advance; refrigerate in jar with tight-fitting lid.)

**2.** For salad, combine lettuce, hearts of palm, avocado, cheese, eggs, tomato, onion and bacon in large bowl. Add dressing; toss to coat.

**MAKES 8 TO 10 SERVINGS (20 CUPS)**

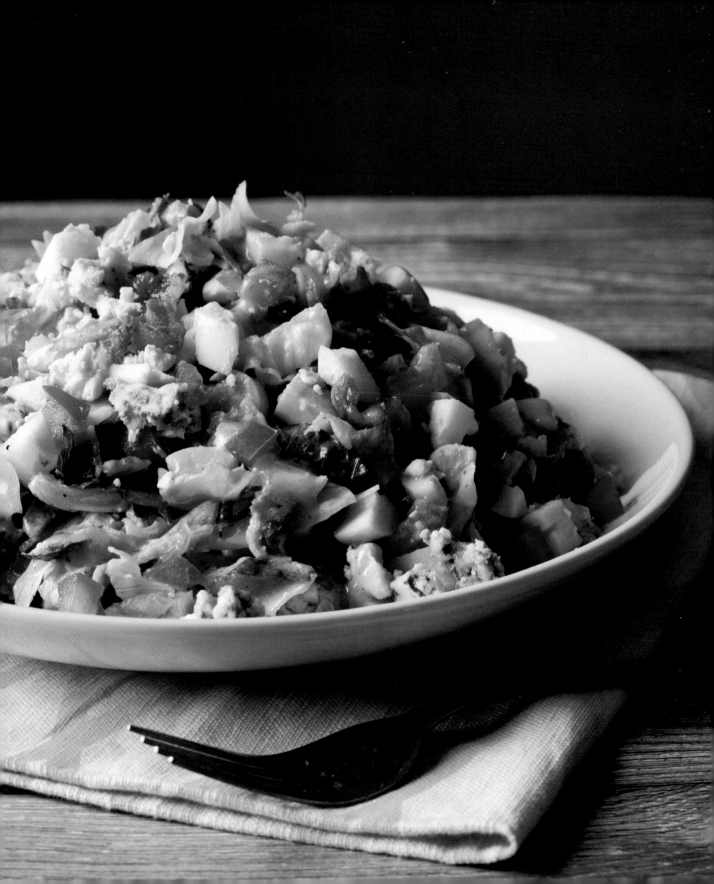

# WEDGE SALAD

## DRESSING

- ¾ **cup mayonnaise**
- ½ **cup buttermilk**
- 1 **cup crumbled blue cheese, divided**
- 1 **clove garlic, minced**
- ½ **teaspoon sugar**
- ⅛ **teaspoon onion powder**
- ⅛ **teaspoon salt**
- ⅛ **teaspoon black pepper**

## SALAD

- 1 **head iceberg lettuce**
- 1 **large tomato, diced (about 1 cup)**
- ½ **small red onion, cut into thin rings**
- 8 **veggie bacon strips, cooked according to package directions and crumbled**

**1.** For dressing, combine mayonnaise, buttermilk, ½ cup cheese, garlic, sugar, onion powder, salt and pepper in food processor or blender; process until smooth.

**2.** For salad, cut lettuce into quarters through stem end; remove stem from each wedge. Place wedges on individual serving plates; top with dressing. Sprinkle with tomato, onion, remaining ½ cup cheese and bacon.

**MAKES 4 SERVINGS**

### TIP

For veggie bacon that looks and acts a little more like the real thing, try frying it like bacon. Heat 2 tablespoons canola oil in a large nonstick skillet over medium heat. Cook veggie bacon strips in batches single layer 1 to 2 minutes per side or until bacon is nicely browned and crispy, adding additional oil as needed. Watch out for oil splatters if your bacon has ice crystals on it.

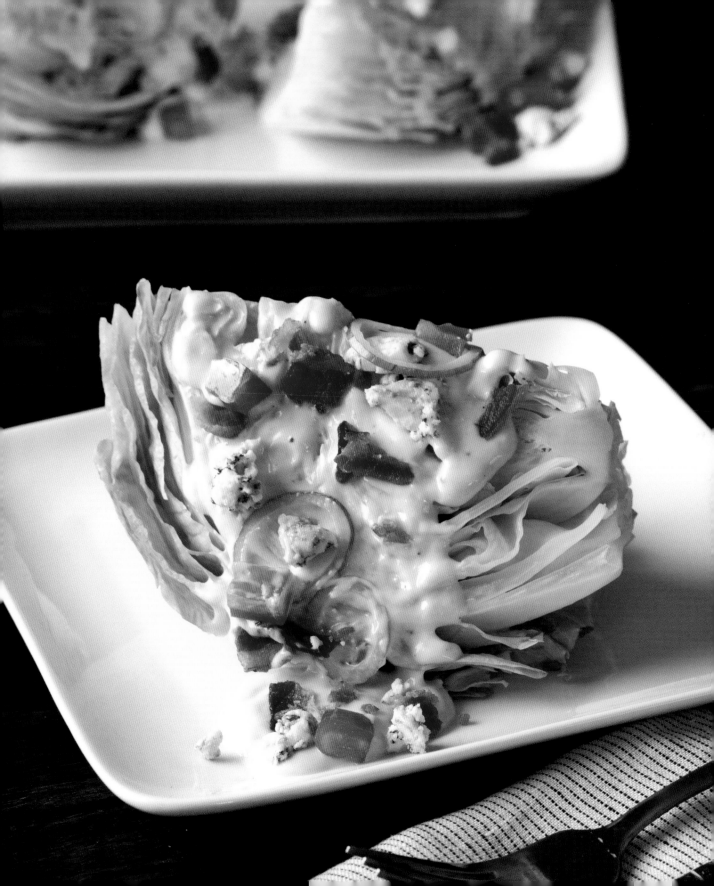

# SPINACH SALAD

## DRESSING

- ¼ **cup balsamic vinegar**
- 1 **clove garlic, minced**
- ½ **teaspoon sugar**
- ¼ **teaspoon salt**
- ⅛ **teaspoon black pepper**
- ¼ **cup olive oil**
- ¼ **cup vegetable oil**

## SALAD

- 8 **cups packed baby spinach**
- 1 **cup diced tomatoes (about 2 medium)**
- 1 **cup drained mandarin oranges**
- 1 **cup glazed pecans***
- ½ **cup crumbled feta cheese**
- ½ **cup diced red onion**
- ½ **cup dried cranberries**
- 1 **can (3 ounces) crispy rice noodles****
- 4 **teaspoons toasted sesame seeds**

*Glazed pecans can be found in the produce section of many supermarkets (with other salad toppings). If unavailable, they can be prepared easily at home. (See Tip.)

**Crispy rice noodles can be found with canned chow mein noodles in the Asian section of the supermarket.

**1.** For dressing, whisk vinegar, garlic, sugar, salt and pepper in medium bowl until blended. Whisk in olive oil and vegetable oil in thin steady stream until well blended.

**2.** Divide spinach among four serving bowls. Top evenly with tomatoes, oranges, pecans, cheese, onion and cranberries. Sprinkle with rice noodles and sesame seeds. Drizzle each salad with 3 tablespoons dressing.

**MAKES 4 SERVINGS**

### TIP

To make glazed pecans, combine 1 cup pecan halves, ¼ cup sugar, 1 tablespoon butter and ½ teaspoon salt in medium skillet; cook and stir over medium heat 5 minutes or until sugar mixture is dark brown and nuts are well coated. Spread on large plate; cool completely. Break into pieces or coarsely chop.

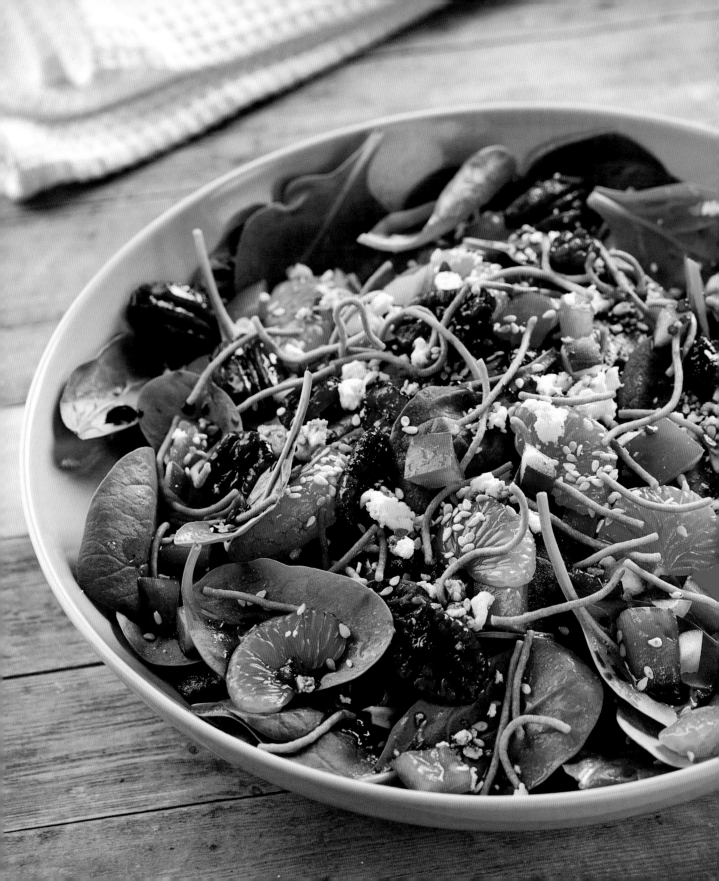

# BBQ CHICKEN SALAD

## DRESSING

- ¾ cup mayonnaise
- ⅓ cup buttermilk
- ¼ cup sour cream
- 1 tablespoon white wine vinegar
- 1 teaspoon sugar
- ¼ teaspoon salt
- ¼ teaspoon garlic powder
- ¼ teaspoon onion powder
- ¼ teaspoon dried parsley flakes
- ¼ teaspoon dried dill weed
- ¼ teaspoon black pepper

## SALAD

- 1 package (8 to 10 ounces) refrigerated meatless chicken strips
- ½ cup barbecue sauce
- 4 cups chopped romaine lettuce
- 4 cups chopped iceberg lettuce
- 2 medium tomatoes, seeded and chopped
- ¾ cup canned or thawed frozen corn, drained
- ¾ cup diced jicama
- ¾ cup (3 ounces) shredded Monterey Jack cheese
- ¼ cup chopped fresh cilantro
- 2 green onions, sliced
- 1 cup crispy tortilla strips*

  *Look for tortilla strips in the produce section with other salad toppings. If they're unavailable, crumble tortilla chips into bite-size pieces.

**1.** For dressing, whisk mayonnaise, buttermilk, sour cream, vinegar, sugar, salt, garlic powder, onion powder, parsley flakes, dill weed and pepper in medium bowl until well blended. Cover and refrigerate until ready to serve.

**2.** For salad, cut meatless chicken strips into ½-inch pieces; place in large bowl. Add barbecue sauce; toss to coat.

**3.** Combine lettuce, tomatoes, corn, jicama, cheese and cilantro in large bowl. Add two thirds of dressing; toss to coat. Add remaining dressing, if necessary. Divide salad among four plates; top with chicken, green onions and tortilla strips.

**MAKES 4 SERVINGS**

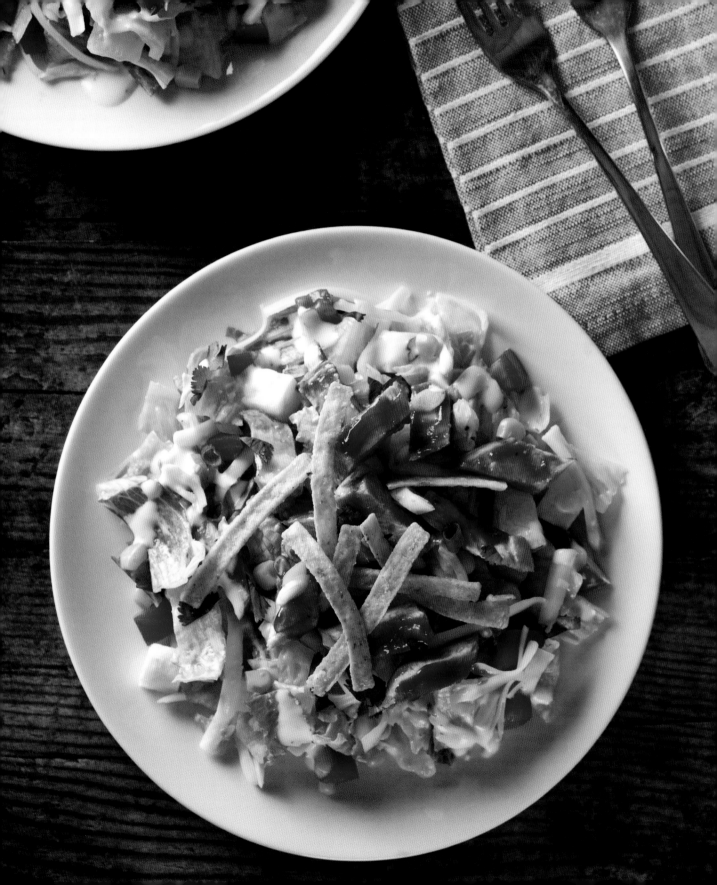

# CABBAGE AND POTATO SALAD WITH CILANTRO-LIME DRESSING

½ cup finely chopped cilantro

2 tablespoons fresh lime juice

2 tablespoons olive oil

2 teaspoons honey

½ teaspoon ground cumin

¼ teaspoon salt

2 cups sliced napa cabbage

2 cups sliced red cabbage

¾ pound baby red potatoes (about 4 potatoes), unpeeled, quartered and cooked

½ cup sliced green onions

2 tablespoons unsalted sunflower kernels

**1.** Whisk cilantro, lime juice, oil, honey, cumin and salt in small bowl until smooth and well blended. Let stand 30 minutes to allow flavors to develop.

**2.** Combine napa cabbage, red cabbage, potatoes and green onions in large bowl; mix well. Add dressing; toss to coat evenly. Sprinkle with sunflower kernels just before serving.

**MAKES 4 SERVINGS**

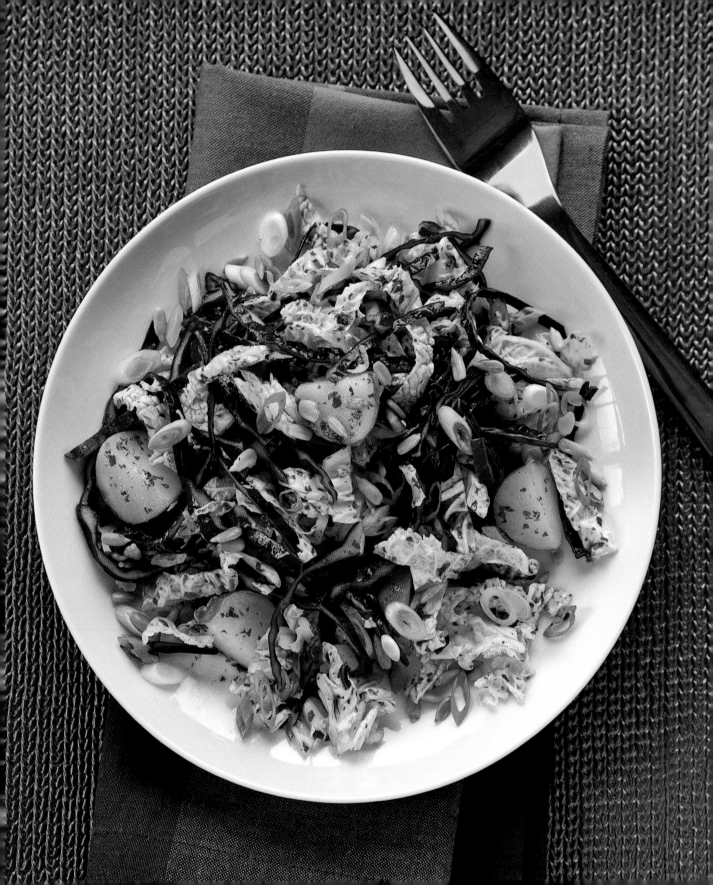

# GREEK SALAD

## SALAD

- 3 medium tomatoes, cut into 8 wedges each and seeds removed
- 1 green bell pepper, cut into 1-inch pieces
- ½ cucumber (8 to 10 inches), quartered lengthwise and sliced crosswise
- ½ red onion, thinly sliced
- ½ cup pitted kalamata olives
- 1 block (8 ounces) feta cheese, cut into ½-inch cubes

## DRESSING

- 6 tablespoons extra virgin olive oil
- 3 tablespoons red wine vinegar
- 1 to 2 cloves garlic, minced
- ¾ teaspoon dried oregano
- ¾ teaspoon salt
- ¼ teaspoon black pepper

**1.** Combine tomatoes, bell pepper, cucumber, onion and olives in large bowl. Top with feta.

**2.** For dressing, whisk oil, vinegar, garlic, oregano, salt and black pepper in medium bowl until well blended. Pour over salad; stir gently to coat.

**MAKES 6 SERVINGS**

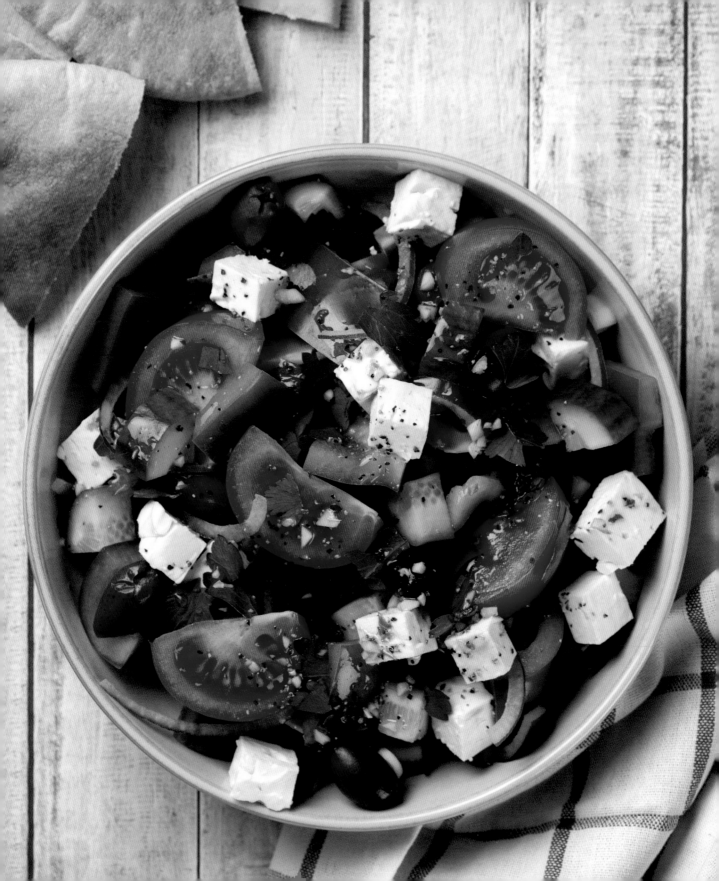

# CHOPPED SALAD WITH CORN BREAD CROUTONS

½ **loaf corn bread (recipe follows)***

1 **large sweet potato, peeled and cut into 1-inch pieces**

5 **tablespoons olive oil, divided**

1½ **teaspoons salt, divided**

3 **tablespoons red wine vinegar**

2 **tablespoons white wine vinegar**

1 **tablespoon maple syrup**

1 **clove garlic, minced**

1 **teaspoon dried mustard**

⅛ **teaspoon dried oregano**

**Pinch red pepper flakes**

½ **cup vegetable oil**

1 **head iceberg lettuce**

1 **cup halved grape tomatoes**

2 **green onions, thinly sliced**

1 **avocado, diced**

½ **cup coarsely chopped smoked almonds**

½ **cup dried cranberries**

*Or purchase corn bread from the bakery of your grocery store or make it from a mix.

**1.** Preheat oven to 400°F. Prepare corn bread. Cool in baking pan at least 10 minutes or cool completely; remove to cutting board. Cut half of corn bread into 1-inch cubes when cool enough to handle. Return to baking dish. *Reduce oven temperature to 350°F.* Bake 12 to 15 minutes or until corn bread cubes are dry and toasted, stirring once.

**2.** Spread sweet potato in 13×9-inch baking pan. Drizzle with 1 tablespoon olive oil and sprinkle with ½ teaspoon salt; toss to coat. Bake 30 to 35 minutes or until browned and tender, stirring once or twice. Cool completely.

**3.** For dressing, whisk vinegars, maple syrup, garlic, mustard, oregano, red pepper flakes and remaining 1 teaspoon salt in medium bowl; whisk in remaining 4 tablespoons olive oil and vegetable oil in thin steady stream.

**4.** Remove outer lettuce leaves and core. Chop lettuce into ½-inch pieces and place in large bowl. Add tomatoes, green onions and half of dressing; mix well. Add sweet potato, avocado, almonds and cranberries; mix well. Taste and add additional dressing, if desired. Add croutons; mix gently.

**MAKES 6 TO 8 SERVINGS**

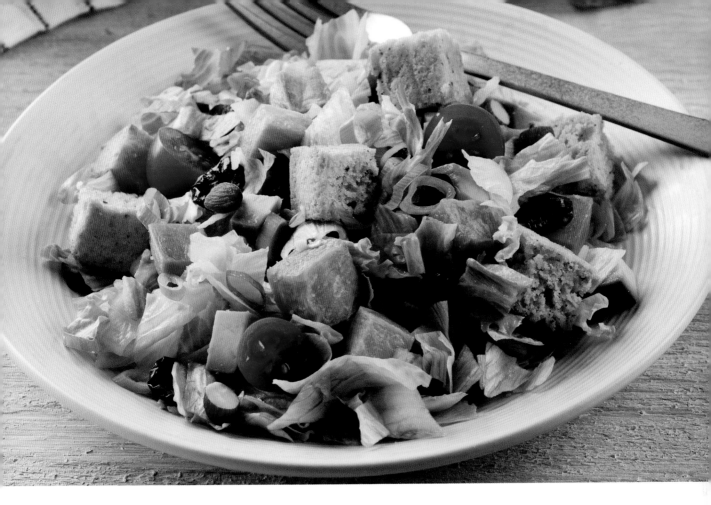

# CORN BREAD

1¼ cups all-purpose flour

¾ cup yellow cornmeal

⅓ cup sugar

2 teaspoons baking powder

1 teaspoon salt

1¼ cups milk or oat milk

¼ cup (½ stick) butter or vegan plant butter, melted

1 egg or flax egg*

*Stir 3 tablespoons boiling water into 1 tablespoon ground flaxseed in small bowl; cool completely.

**1.** Preheat oven to 400°F. Spray 8-inch square baking dish or pan with nonstick cooking spray.

**2.** Combine flour, cornmeal, sugar, baking powder and salt in large bowl; mix well. Beat milk, butter and egg in medium bowl until well blended. Add to flour mixture; stir just until dry ingredients are moistened. Pour batter into prepared baking dish.

**3.** Bake 25 minutes or until golden brown and toothpick inserted into center comes out clean.

# BROCCOLI-RAISIN SALAD

4 cups small fresh
   broccoli florets

½ cup golden raisins or
   dried cranberries

½ medium red onion,
   finely chopped

¼ cup dry-roasted
   sunflower seeds

¼ cup mayonnaise

2 tablespoons milk

1 tablespoon sugar

2 teaspoons cider
   vinegar

½ teaspoon salt

   Black pepper

**1.** Combine broccoli, raisins, onion and sunflower seeds in large bowl.

**2.** Whisk mayonnaise, milk, sugar, vinegar and salt in medium bowl; season with pepper. Pour over broccoli mixture; mix well. Serve immediately or cover and refrigerate until ready to serve.

**MAKES 4 TO 6 SERVINGS**

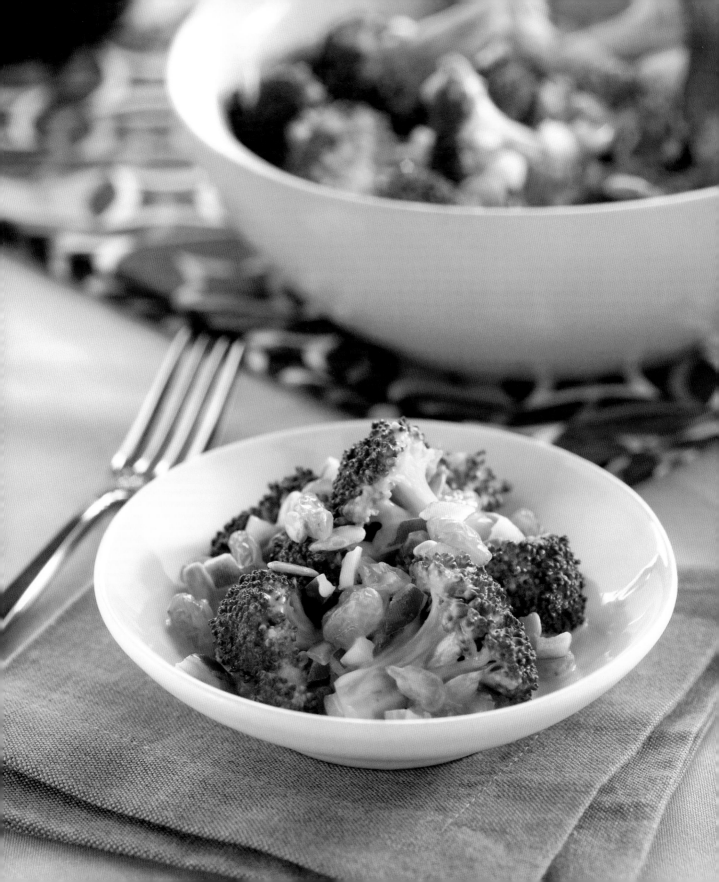

# CAULIFLOWER CHOPPED SALAD

½ cup red wine vinegar

¼ cup olive oil

1 teaspoon salt

1 teaspoon honey

1 teaspoon Dijon mustard

½ teaspoon dried oregano

1 clove garlic, minced

¼ teaspoon black pepper

2 cups small cauliflower florets (½ inch)

1 head iceberg lettuce, chopped

1 container (4 ounces) crumbled blue cheese

1 pint grape tomatoes, halved *or* 1 cup finely chopped tomatoes

½ cup finely chopped red onion

2 green onions, finely chopped

1 avocado, diced

**1.** For cauliflower, whisk vinegar, oil, salt, honey, mustard, oregano, garlic and pepper in medium bowl. Add cauliflower; stir to coat. Cover and refrigerate several hours or overnight.

**2.** For salad, combine lettuce, blue cheese, tomatoes, red onion and green onions in large bowl; toss to coat. Remove cauliflower from marinade using slotted spoon; place on salad. Whisk marinade; pour over salad and toss to coat. Top with avocado; mix gently.

**MAKES 8 SERVINGS**

**TIP**

Vegan Swaps: Replace honey with maple syrup and skip the cheese.

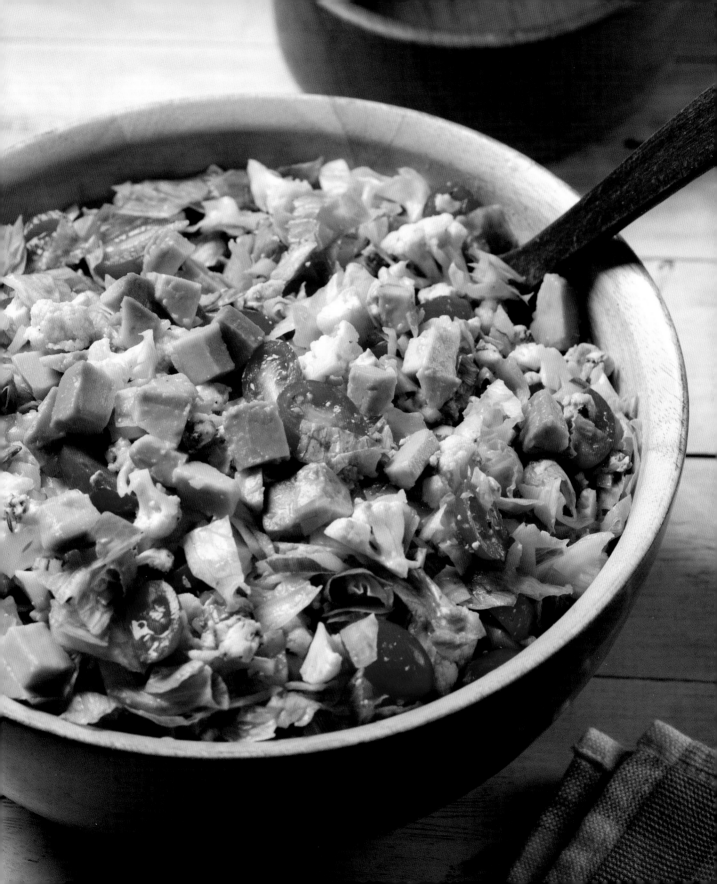

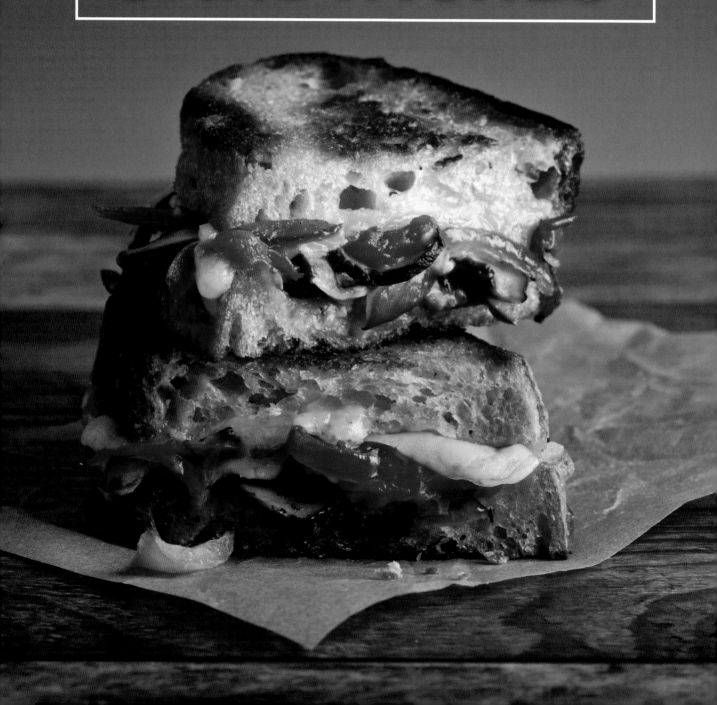

# CHAPTER 3
# SANDWICHES

# TUSCAN PORTOBELLO MELT

1 **portobello mushroom cap, thinly sliced**

½ **small red onion, thinly sliced**

½ **cup grape tomatoes**

1 **tablespoon olive oil**

1 **teaspoon balsamic vinegar**

⅛ **teaspoon salt**

⅛ **teaspoon dried thyme**

⅛ **teaspoon black pepper**

2 **tablespoons butter, softened and divided**

4 **slices sourdough bread**

2 **slices provolone cheese**

2 **teaspoons Dijon mustard**

2 **slices Monterey Jack cheese**

**1.** Preheat broiler. Combine mushroom, onion and tomatoes in small baking pan. Drizzle with oil and vinegar; sprinkle with salt, thyme and pepper. Toss to coat. Spread vegetables in single layer in pan.

**2.** Broil 6 minutes or until vegetables are softened and browned, stirring once.

**3.** Heat medium skillet over medium heat. Spread 1 tablespoon butter over one side of each bread slice. Place buttered side down in skillet; cook 2 minutes or until bread is toasted. Transfer bread to cutting board, toasted sides up.

**4.** Place provolone cheese on 2 bread slices; spread mustard over cheese. Top with vegetables, Monterey Jack cheese and remaining bread slices, toasted sides down. Spread remaining 1 tablespoon butter on outside of sandwiches. Cook in same skillet over medium heat 5 minutes or until bread is toasted and cheese is melted, turning once.

**MAKES 2 SERVINGS**

# HAVARTI AND ONION SANDWICHES

1½ teaspoons olive oil

⅓ cup thinly sliced red onion

4 slices pumpernickel bread

½ cup prepared coleslaw

6 ounces dill havarti cheese, cut into slices

**1.** Heat oil in large skillet over medium heat. Add onion; cook and stir 5 minutes or until tender. Layer onion, cheese and coleslaw on 2 bread slices; top with remaining 2 bread slices.

**2.** Heat same skillet over medium heat. Add sandwiches; press down with spatula or weigh down with small plate. Cook 4 to 5 minutes on each side or until cheese is melted and sandwiches are browned.

**MAKES 2 SANDWICHES**

TIP

For this sandwich (and pretty much any other toasted sandwich), you can use a panini press, electric indoor countertop grill or grill pan.

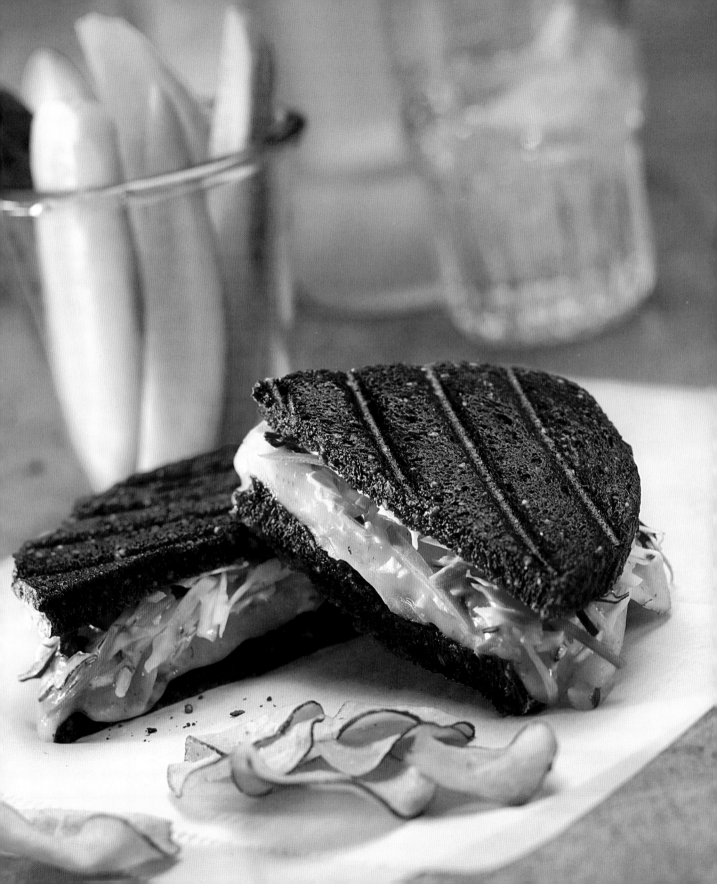

# CAULIFLOWER TACOS WITH CHIPOTLE CREMA

**Pickled Red Onions (recipe follows) or sliced red onion**

1 **package (8 ounces) sliced cremini mushrooms**

4 **tablespoons olive oil, divided**

1¾ **teaspoons salt, divided**

1 **head cauliflower**

1 **teaspoon ground cumin**

½ **teaspoon dried oregano**

¼ **teaspoon ground coriander**

¼ **teaspoon ground cinnamon**

¼ **teaspoon black pepper**

½ **cup vegan sour cream**

2 **teaspoons lime juice**

½ **teaspoon chipotle chili powder**

½ **cup vegetarian refried beans**

8 **taco-size flour or corn tortillas**

**Chopped fresh cilantro (optional)**

**1.** Prepare pickled red onions. Preheat oven to 400°F. Toss mushrooms with 1 tablespoon oil and ¼ teaspoon salt in large bowl. Spread on small baking sheet.

**2.** Break cauliflower into florets; cut into 1-inch pieces. Place in same large bowl. Add remaining 3 tablespoons olive oil, 1 teaspoon salt, cumin, oregano, coriander, cinnamon and black pepper; mix well. Spread on sheet pan in single layer.

**3.** Roast cauliflower about 40 minutes or until browned and tender, stirring a few times. Roast mushrooms 20 minutes or until dry and browned, stirring once.

**4.** For crema, combine sour cream, lime juice, chipotle and remaining ½ teaspoon salt in small bowl.

**5.** For each taco, spread 1 tablespoon beans over tortilla; spread 1 teaspoon crema over beans. Top with about 3 mushroom slices and ¼ cup cauliflower. Top with cilantro and red onions, if desired. Fold in half.

**MAKES 8 TACOS (4 SERVINGS)**

### PICKLED RED ONIONS

Thinly slice 1 small red onion; place in large glass jar. Add ¼ cup white wine vinegar or distilled white vinegar, 2 tablespoons water, 1 teaspoon sugar and 1 teaspoon salt. Seal jar; shake well. Refrigerate at least 1 hour or up to 1 week. Makes about ½ cup.

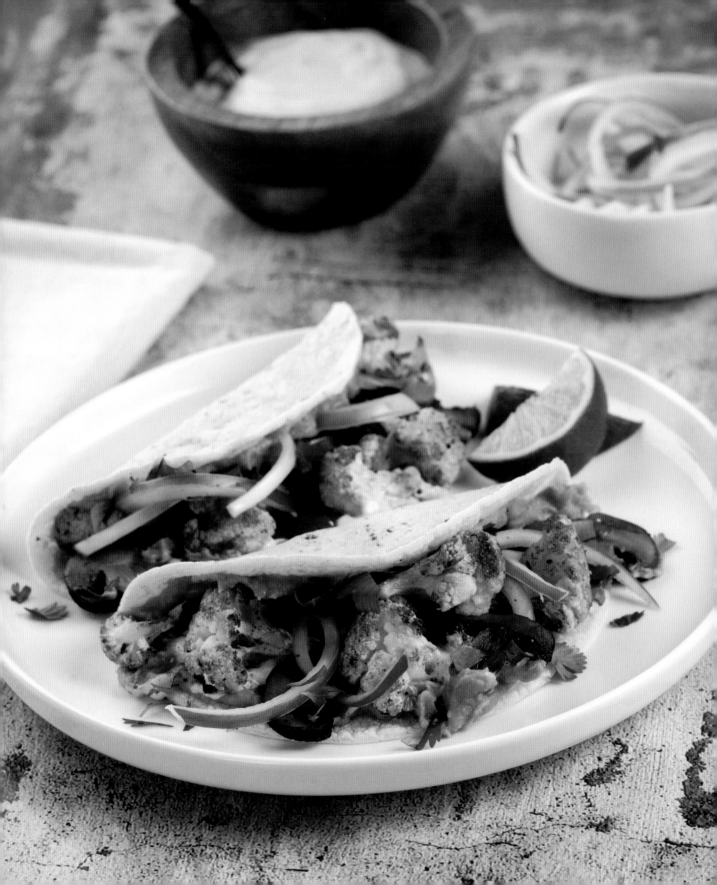

# MEATLESS SLOPPY JOES

1 tablespoon olive oil

2 cups thinly sliced onions

2 cups chopped green bell peppers

2 cloves garlic, finely chopped

2 tablespoons ketchup

1 tablespoon yellow mustard

1 can (about 15 ounces) kidney beans, rinsed, drained and mashed

1 can (8 ounces) tomato sauce

1 teaspoon chili powder

2 tablespoons cider vinegar

4 sandwich rolls

**1.** Heat oil in large skillet over medium heat. Add onions, bell peppers and garlic; cook and stir 5 minutes or until vegetables are tender. Stir in ketchup and mustard.

**2.** Add beans, tomato sauce and chili powder. Reduce heat to medium-low. Cook 5 minutes or until thickened, stirring frequently. Stir in vinegar. Serve on sandwich rolls.

**MAKES 4 SERVINGS**

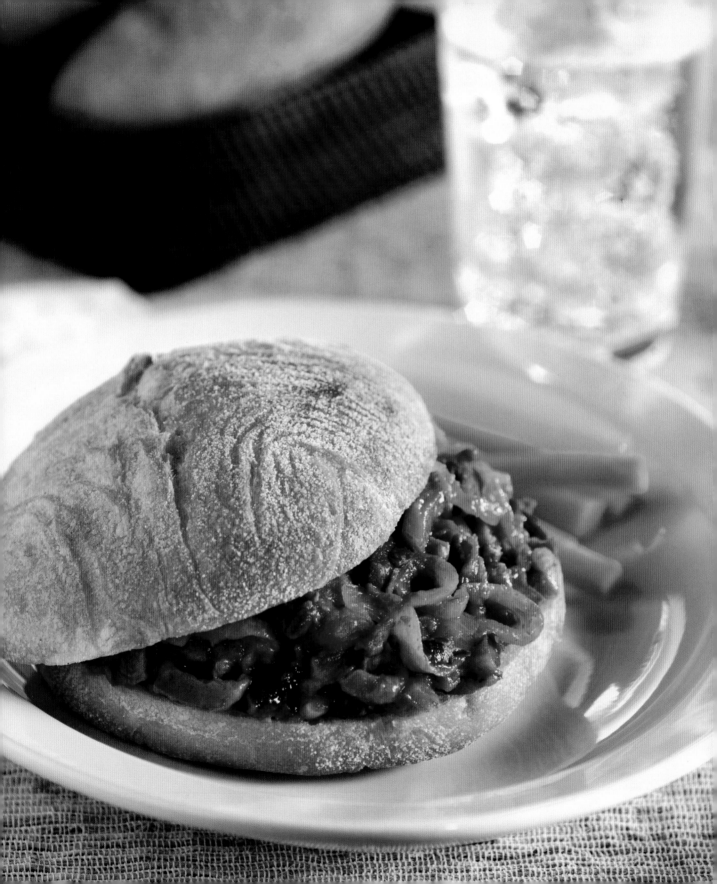

# TOMATO AND CHEESE MELTS

2 tablespoons
  mayonnaise

2 teaspoons prepared
  pesto

4 slices whole grain
  bread

4 tomato slices (about
  ¼ inch thick)

4 thin cucumber slices
  (⅛ inch thick and
  3 inches long)

2 slices mozzarella
  cheese

**1.** Combine mayonnaise and pesto in small bowl; spread evenly on 2 bread slices. Top with tomato, cucumber, cheese and remaining bread slices.

**2.** Spray grill pan or large skillet with nonstick cooking spray; heat over medium heat. Cook sandwiches about 3 to 4 minutes per side or until lightly browned; reduce heat if toasting too quickly. Cover during last 2 minutes of cooking to melt cheese. Cut sandwiches in half.

**MAKES 2 SERVINGS**

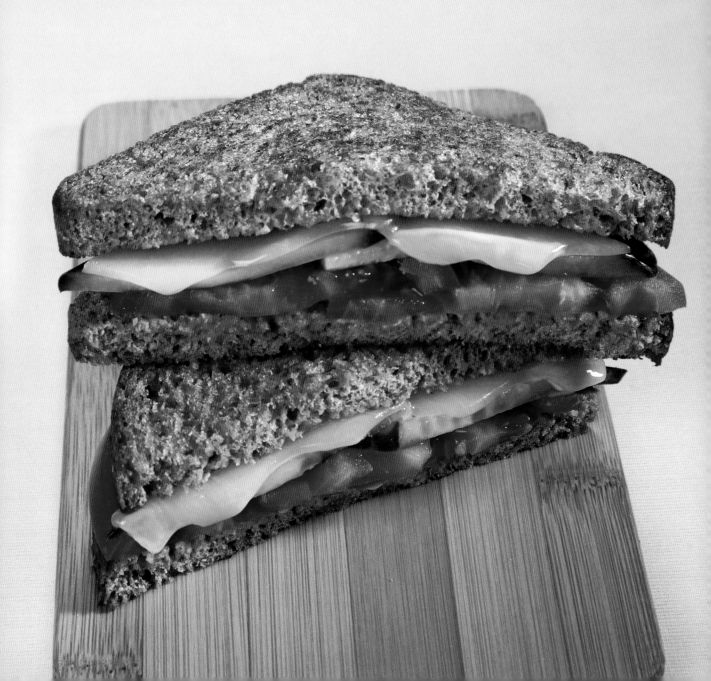

# CHICKPEA SALAD

1 can (15 ounces) chickpeas, rinsed and drained

1 stalk celery, chopped

1 dill pickle, chopped (about ½ cup)

¼ cup finely chopped red or yellow onion

⅓ cup mayonnaise (regular or vegan)

1 teaspoon lemon juice

¼ teaspoon salt

Black pepper

Whole grain bread

Lettuce and tomato slices

1. Place chickpeas in medium bowl. Coarsely mash with potato masher, leaving some beans whole.

2. Add celery, pickle and onion; stir to mix. Add mayonnaise and lemon juice; mix well. Taste and add ¼ teaspoon salt or more, if desired. Season with pepper; mix well. Serve on bread with lettuce and tomato.

**MAKES 2 CUPS (4 TO 6 SERVINGS)**

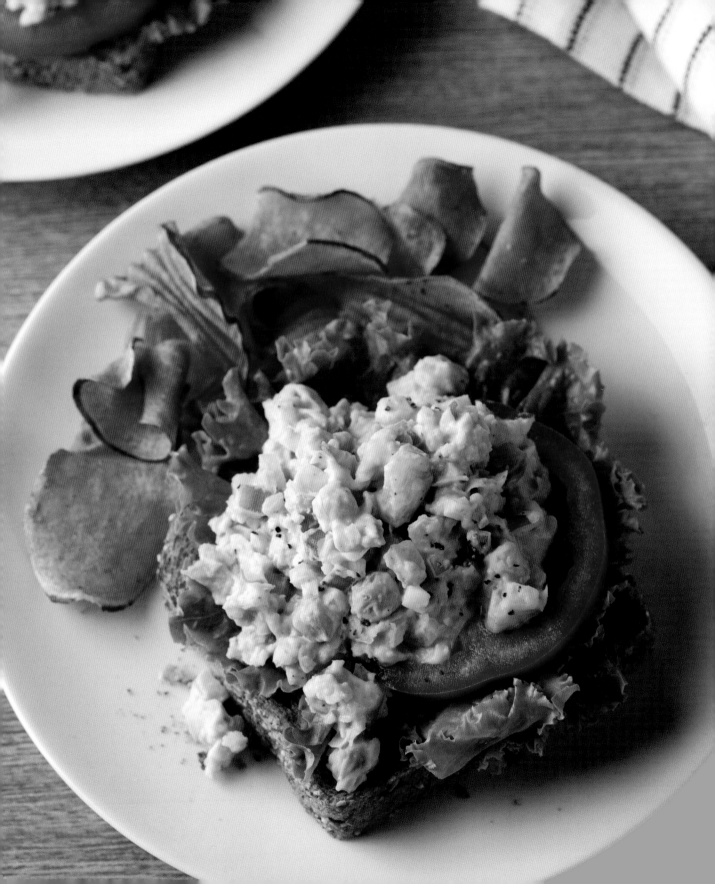

# PEAR GORGONZOLA MELTS

**4 ounces creamy
Gorgonzola cheese
(do not use crumbled
blue cheese)**

**8 slices walnut raisin
bread**

**2 pears, cored and sliced**

**½ cup baby spinach**

**2 tablespoons softened
butter**

**1.** Spread cheese evenly on 4 bread slices; layer with pears and spinach. Top with remaining bread slices. Spread butter on outsides of sandwiches.

**2.** Heat large nonstick skillet over medium heat. Add sandwiches; cook 4 to 5 minutes per side or until cheese is melted and sandwiches are golden brown.

**MAKES 4 SERVINGS**

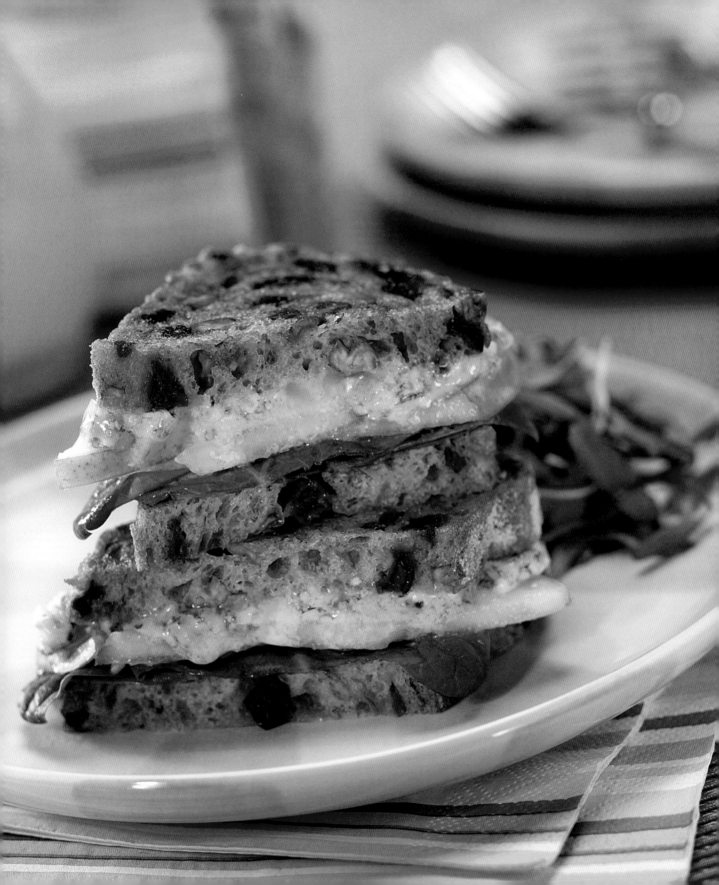

# DOUBLE DECKER TACOS

2 tablespoons all-purpose flour

2 teaspoons chili powder

1 teaspoon dried minced onion

¾ teaspoon paprika

½ teaspoon salt

½ teaspoon garlic powder

¼ teaspoon sugar

1 pound refrigerated plant-based ground meatless product *or* 1 package (10 ounces) frozen meatless crumbles

⅔ cup water

8 taco shells

8 mini (5-inch) flour tortillas*

2 cups refried beans, warmed

2 cups shredded romaine lettuce

1 cup chopped tomato

1 cup (4 ounces) shredded Cheddar cheese

Sour cream

*Mini tortillas are also labeled as street tacos.

**1.** Preheat oven to 350°F. Combine flour, chili powder, onion, paprika, salt, garlic powder and sugar in small bowl; mix well.

**2.** Cook ground meatless product in large skillet over medium-high heat until browned, stirring frequently to break into small crumbles. Drain fat and excess liquid from skillet. Add seasoning mixture; cook and stir 2 minutes. Stir in water; bring to a simmer. Reduce heat to medium; cook about 10 minutes or until most of liquid has evaporated.

**3.** Meanwhile, heat taco shells in oven about 5 minutes or until warm.

**4.** Wrap tortillas in damp paper towel; microwave on HIGH 25 to 35 seconds or until warm. Spread each tortilla with ¼ cup refried beans, leaving ¼-inch border around edges. Wrap flour tortillas around taco shells, pressing gently to seal together.

**5.** Fill taco shells with meatless mixture. Top with lettuce, tomato and cheese. Serve with sour cream.

**MAKES 8 TACOS**

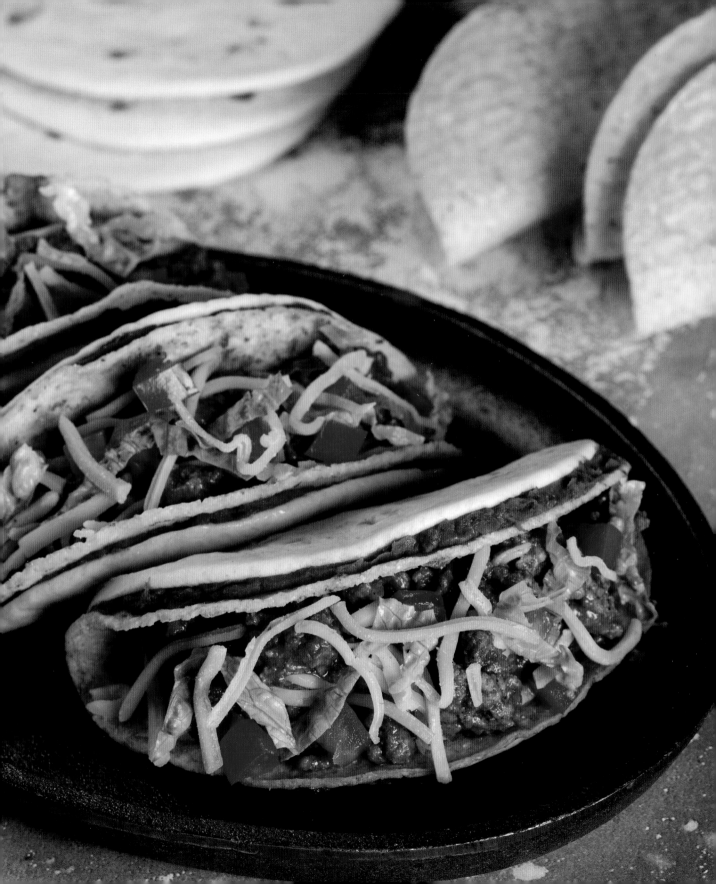

# GRILLED PORTOBELLO SANDWICHES

2 tablespoons extra virgin olive oil

1½ tablespoons balsamic vinegar

1 tablespoon coarse grain Dijon mustard

1 tablespoon water

1 teaspoon dried oregano

1 clove garlic, minced

½ teaspoon black pepper

¼ teaspoon salt

4 large portobello mushroom caps, wiped with damp towel, gills and stems removed

8 slices multigrain Italian bread (8 ounces)

¼ cup crumbled blue cheese

2 to 3 ounces spring greens

1. Combine oil, vinegar, mustard, water, oregano, garlic, pepper and salt in medium bowl. Place mushrooms in single layer on baking sheet or large plate. Brush 2 tablespoons dressing over mushrooms; set aside remaining dressing. Let mushrooms stand 30 minutes.

2. Spray grill pan with nonstick cooking spray; heat over medium-high heat. Spray both sides of bread slices with cooking spray. Grill bread 1 minute per side, pressing down with spatula to flatten slightly. Set aside.

3. Grill mushrooms 3 to 4 minutes per side or until tender. Place each mushroom on 1 slice of bread. Sprinkle with blue cheese.

4. Combine spring greens and reserved dressing. Arrange spring greens on top of mushrooms; top with remaining bread slices.

**MAKES 4 SERVINGS**

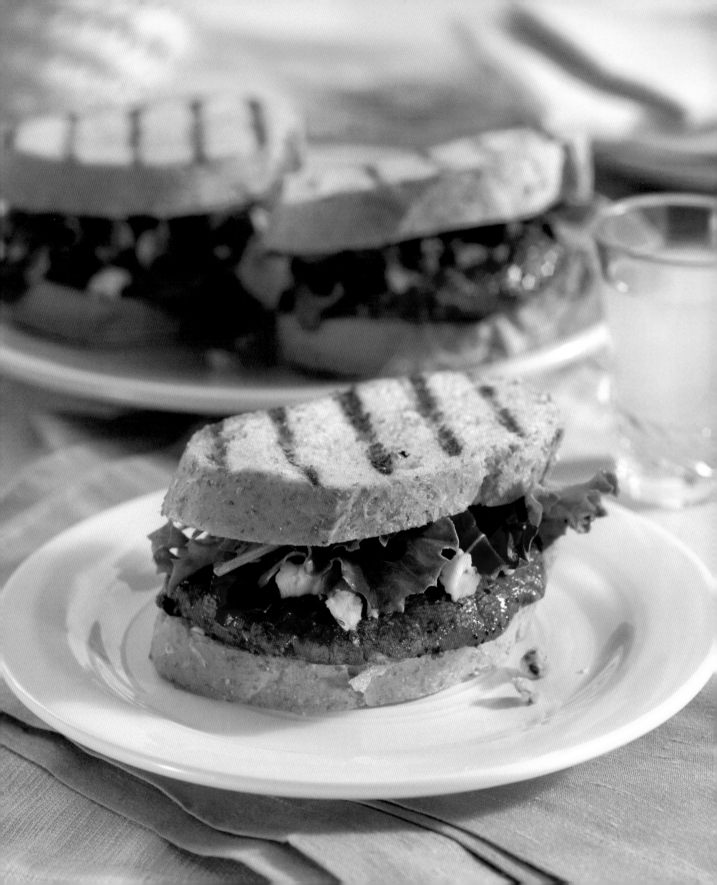

# BLACK BEAN BURGERS WITH SPICY MAYO

5 whole wheat hamburger buns, split, divided

1 can (about 15 ounces) black beans, rinsed and drained

½ cup (2 ounces) shredded Cheddar cheese or Mexican blend cheese

2 egg whites

2 green onions, sliced

1 teaspoon chili powder

1 teaspoon dried oregano

½ teaspoon garlic salt

1 tablespoon canola oil

2 tablespoons mayonnaise

¾ teaspoon chipotle hot pepper sauce

Lettuce leaves and tomato slices

**1.** Tear 1 hamburger bun into pieces; place in bowl of food processor. Pulse until coarse crumbs form. Transfer to medium bowl (there should be at least 1 cup bread crumbs).

**2.** Add black beans, cheese, egg whites, green onions, chili powder, oregano and garlic salt to food processor. Process until mixture is thick and finely ground, scraping down sides of bowl once. Add mixture to bread crumbs in bowl; mix well.

**3.** Heat oil in large nonstick skillet over medium heat. Use ½-cup measuring cup to scoop bean mixture. Drop 4 mounds into skillet; press down to form 3½- to 4-inch patties. Cook 4 minutes per side or until browned. Lightly toast remaining hamburger buns, if desired.

**4.** Combine mayonnaise and hot pepper sauce in small bowl. Serve patties in buns with mayonnaise mixture, lettuce and tomato.

**MAKES 4 SERVINGS**

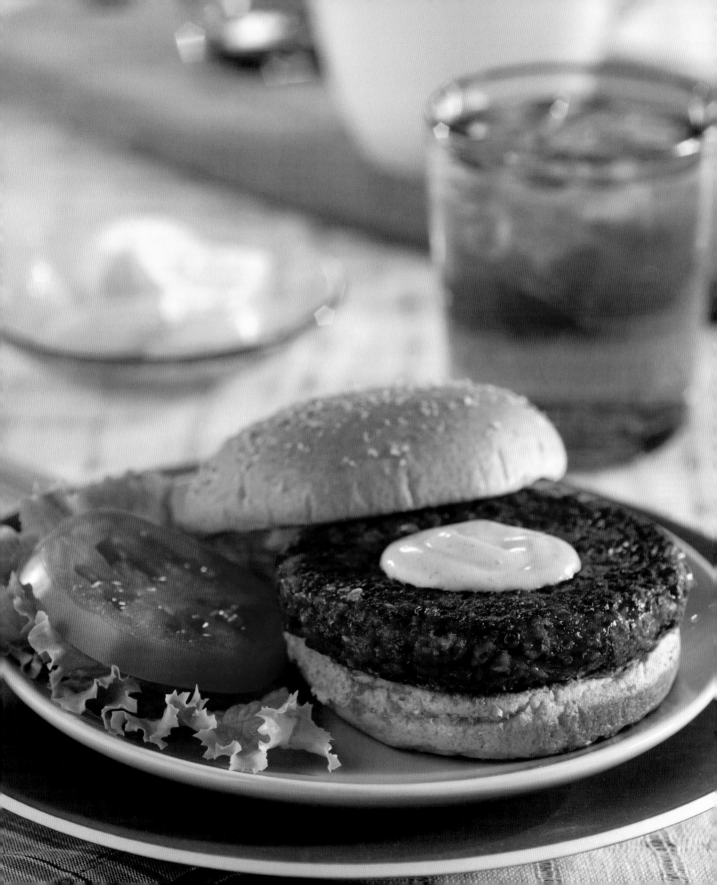

# BARBECUE CAULIFLOWER CALZONES

1 head cauliflower, cut
    into florets and thinly
    sliced

2 tablespoons olive oil

Salt and black pepper

¾ cup barbecue sauce

1 can (about 13 ounces)
    pizza dough

½ yellow onion, chopped

1 cup (4 ounces)
    shredded mozzarella
    cheese

Ranch or blue cheese
    dressing

1. Preheat oven to 400°F.

2. Spread cauliflower on sheet pan; drizzle with oil and season lightly with salt and pepper. Toss to coat; spread in single layer.

3. Roast 30 minutes or until cauliflower is browned and very tender, stirring once. Transfer to medium bowl; stir in barbecue sauce.

4. Unroll pizza dough onto cutting board. Stretch into 11×17-inch rectangle; cut into quarters. Place one fourth of onion on half of each piece of dough. Top with one fourth of cauliflower and ¼ cup cheese. Bring dough over filling; roll and pinch edges to seal. Place on baking sheet. Spray with nonstick cooking spray or brush with oil to help crust brown.

5. Bake 10 minutes or until golden brown. Serve with ranch dressing.

**MAKES 4 SERVINGS**

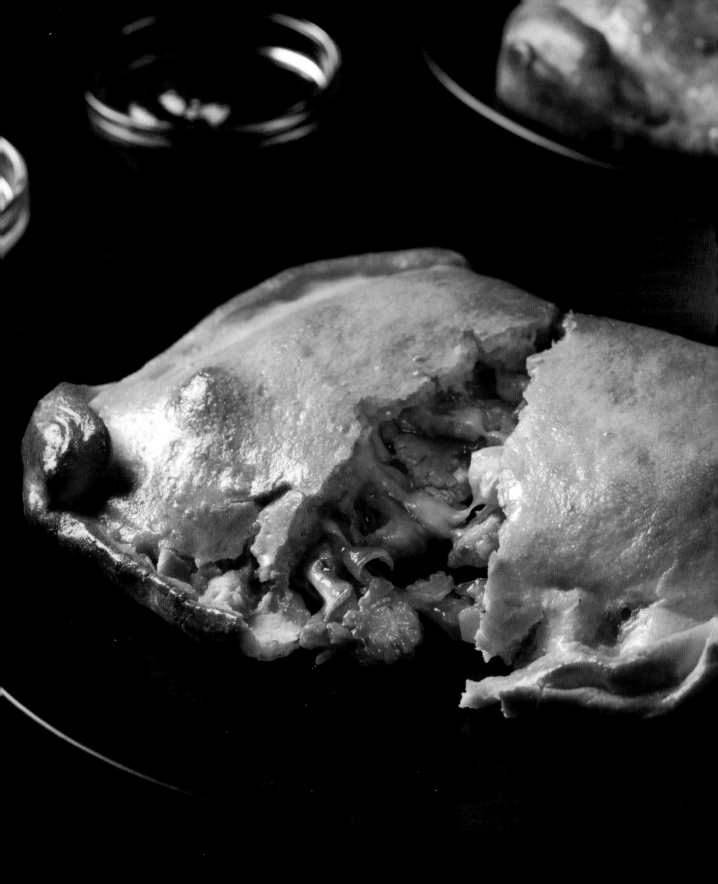

# WILD MUSHROOM TOFU BURGERS

3 teaspoons olive oil, divided

1 package (8 ounces) cremini mushrooms, coarsely chopped

½ medium onion, roughly chopped

1 clove garlic, minced

7 ounces extra firm tofu, crumbled and frozen

1 cup old-fashioned oats

⅓ cup finely chopped walnuts

1 egg

½ teaspoon salt

½ teaspoon onion powder

¼ teaspoon dried thyme

6 English muffins, split and toasted

Lettuce, tomato and red onion slices (optional)

1. Heat 1 teaspoon oil in large nonstick skillet over medium heat. Add mushrooms, onion and garlic; cook and stir 10 minutes or until mushrooms have released most of their liquid. Remove from heat; cool slightly.

2. Combine mushroom mixture, tofu, oats, walnuts, egg, salt, onion powder and thyme in food processor or blender; process until combined. (Some tofu pieces may remain). Shape mixture by ⅓-cupfuls into six patties.

3. Heat 1 teaspoon oil in same skillet over medium-low heat. Working in batches, cook patties 5 minutes per side or until browned, adding remaining 1 teaspoon oil between batches.

4. Serve burgers on English muffins with lettuce, tomato and red onion, if desired.

**MAKES 6 SERVINGS**

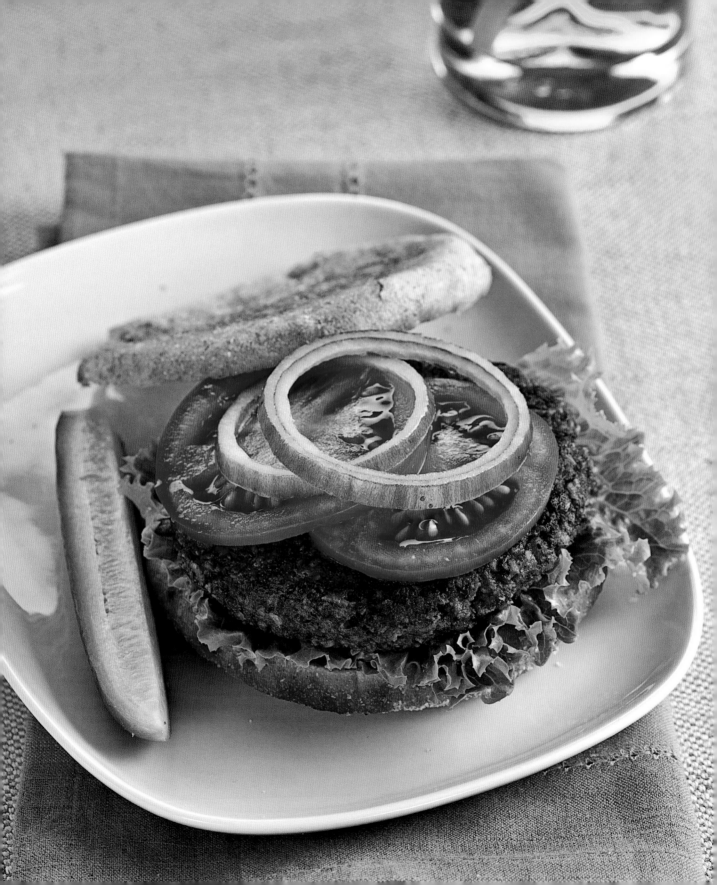

# CHORIZO QUESADILLAS

1 package (9 ounces) vegetarian chorizo

1 cup coarsely chopped cauliflower

1 small onion, finely chopped

12 (6-inch) flour tortillas

1½ cups (6 ounces) chihuahua cheese

6 teaspoons vegetable oil

Salsa, guacamole and sour cream

**1.** Heat medium skillet over medium-high heat. Add chorizo, cauliflower and onion; cook and stir 10 to 12 minutes or until cauliflower is tender. Transfer to bowl. Wipe out skillet.

**2.** Spread ¼ cup chorizo mixture onto each of 6 tortillas. Top with ¼ cup cheese and remaining tortillas.

**3.** Heat 1 teaspoon oil in same skillet over medium-high heat. Add one quesadilla; cook 2 to 3 minutes per side or until well browned and cheese is melted. Repeat with remaining oil and quesadillas. Cut into wedges; serve with salsa, guacamole and sour cream.

**MAKES 6 SERVINGS**

TIP

To keep cooked quesadillas warm, arrange on a baking sheet and place in a preheated 200°F oven until all the quesadillas are cooked and ready to serve.

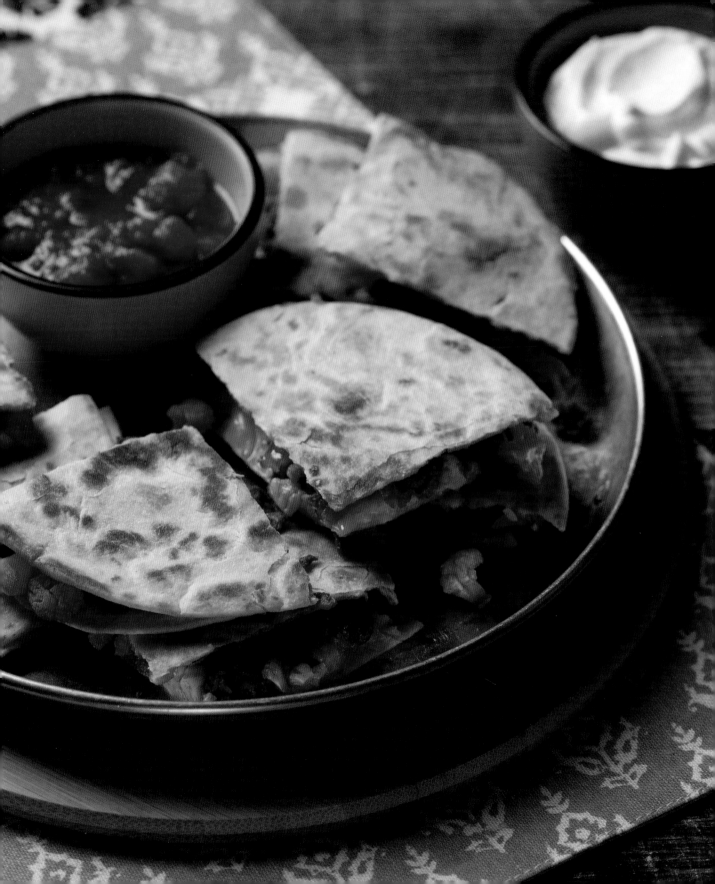

# HEARTY VEGGIE SANDWICH

1 pound cremini mushrooms, stemmed and thinly sliced (⅛-inch slices)

2 tablespoons olive oil, divided

¾ teaspoon salt, divided

¼ teaspoon black pepper

1 medium zucchini, diced (¼-inch pieces, about 2 cups)

3 tablespoons butter, softened

8 slices artisan whole grain bread

¼ cup prepared pesto

¼ cup mayonnaise

2 cups packed baby spinach

4 slices (about 1 ounce each) mozzarella cheese

**1.** Preheat oven to 350°F. Combine mushrooms, 1 tablespoon oil, ½ teaspoon salt and pepper in medium bowl; toss to coat. Spread on large rimmed baking sheet. Roast 20 minutes or until mushrooms are dark brown and dry, stirring after 10 minutes. Cool on baking sheet.

**2.** Meanwhile, heat remaining 1 tablespoon oil in large skillet over medium heat. Add zucchini and remaining ¼ teaspoon salt; cook and stir 5 minutes or until zucchini is tender and lightly browned. Transfer to bowl; wipe out skillet with paper towels.

**3.** Spread butter over one side of each bread slice. Turn over slices. Spread pesto over 4 slices; spread mayonnaise over remaining 4 slices. Top pesto-covered slices evenly with mushrooms, then spinach, zucchini and cheese. Top with remaining bread slices, mayonnaise side down.

**4.** Heat same skillet over medium heat. Add sandwiches; cover and cook 2 minutes per side or until bread is toasted, spinach is slightly wilted and cheese is beginning to melt. Cut sandwiches in half; serve immediately.

**MAKES 4 SERVINGS**

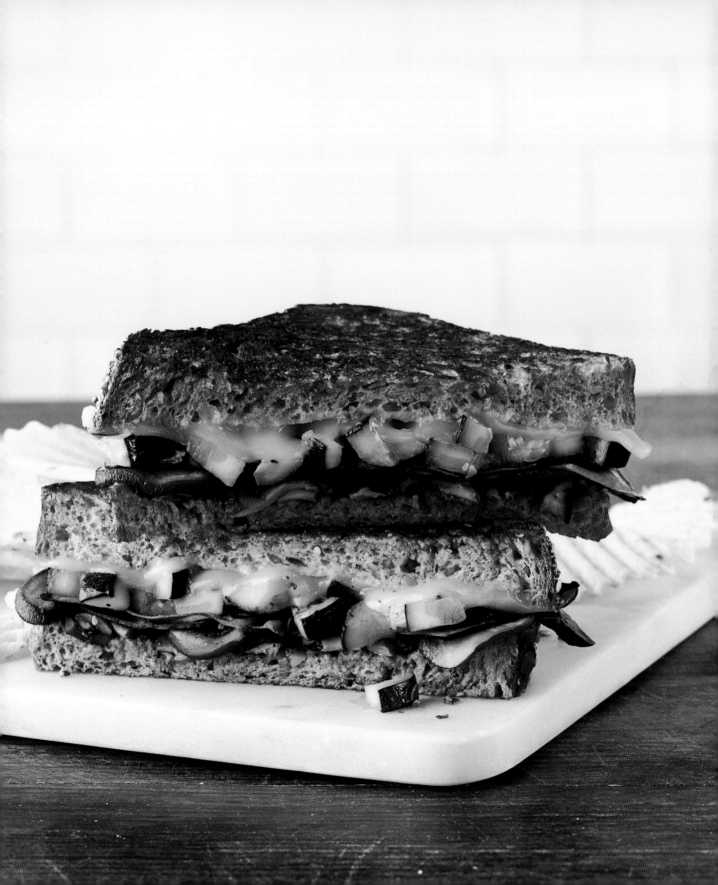

# LAMB-STYLE NAAN AND RAITA SANDWICH

1 tablespoon olive oil

1 red onion, diced

1 pound refrigerated plant-based ground meatless product

1¼ teaspoons minced garlic, divided

1 tablespoon tomato paste

1 teaspoon ground cumin

½ teaspoon ground coriander

1½ teaspoons kosher salt, divided

½ cup diced cucumber

¾ cup plain Greek yogurt or sour cream

2 tablespoons chopped fresh cilantro

4 pieces of naan bread, warmed or toasted

**1.** Heat oil in large skillet over medium heat. Add onion; cook and stir 8 to 10 minutes or until softened. Transfer to small bowl.

**2.** Cook meatless product in same skillet over medium-high heat about 8 minutes or until well browned, stirring to break into crumbles. Add 1 teaspoon garlic, tomato paste, cumin, coriander and 1 teaspoon salt; cook 1 minute, stirring constantly. Add onion; cook 1 minute.

**3.** Combine cucumber, yogurt, remaining ¼ teaspoon garlic, cilantro and remaining ½ teaspoon salt in medium bowl.

**4.** Divide meatless mixture evenly among warmed naan; top with raita. Serve immediately.

**MAKES 4 SERVINGS**

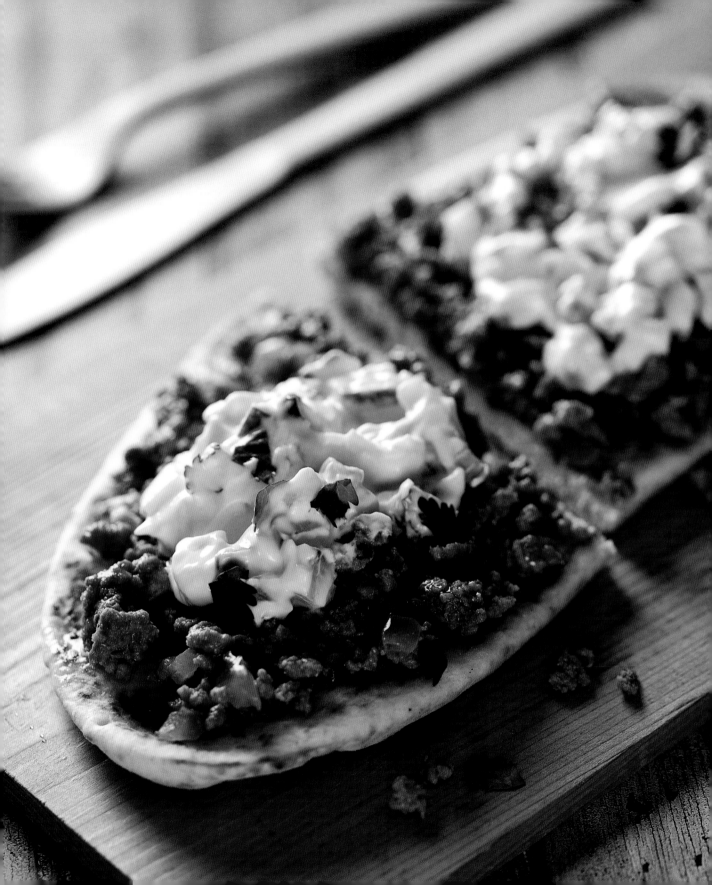

# MOZZARELLA IN CARROZZA

2 eggs

⅓ cup milk

¼ teaspoon salt

⅛ teaspoon black pepper

8 slices country Italian bread

6 ounces fresh mozzarella, cut into ¼-inch slices

8 oil-packed sun-dried tomatoes, drained and cut into strips

8 to 12 fresh basil leaves, torn

1½ tablespoons olive oil

1. Whisk eggs, milk, salt and pepper in shallow bowl or baking dish until well blended.

2. Place 4 bread slices on work surface. Top with mozzarella, sun-dried tomatoes, basil and remaining bread slices.

3. Heat oil in large skillet over medium heat. Dip sandwiches in egg mixture, turning and pressing to coat completely. Place sandwiches in skillet; cook 5 minutes per side or until golden brown. Cut into strips or squares.

**MAKES 4 SERVINGS**

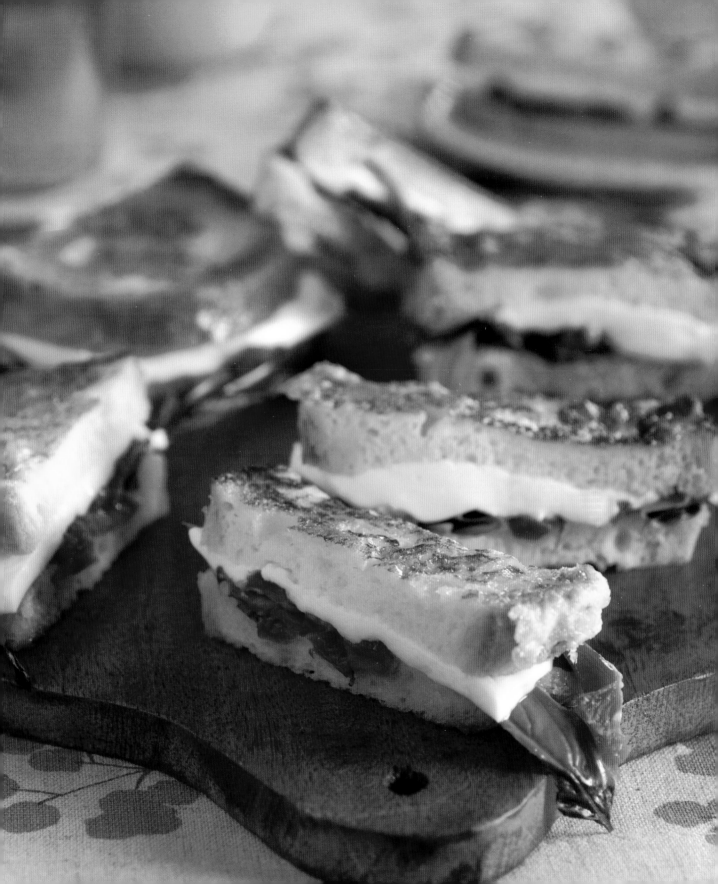

# GARDEN BRUSCHETTA

1 medium zucchini, cut into ¼-inch-thick diagonal slices

1 large shallot or small red onion, thinly sliced

1 teaspoon olive oil

¼ teaspoon black pepper

2 slices artisan whole wheat bread

1 clove garlic, crushed

2 small plum tomatoes, thinly sliced

¼ teaspoon dried oregano, divided

1 tablespoon chopped fresh basil

3 jumbo pimiento-stuffed olives, thinly sliced

3 tablespoons shredded Parmesan cheese, divided

**1.** Preheat grill to medium-high heat. Place zucchini and shallot slices in grill basket or vegetable grate. Brush with oil and sprinkle with pepper. Grill 3 to 5 minutes per side, or until tender and lightly browned. Remove from heat. (Or cook vegetables in 1 teaspoon oil in large skillet over medium-high heat until tender.)

**2.** Rub bread slices with garlic; discard garlic. Grill bread 1 to 2 minutes or until lightly browned. Or toast bread slices under broiler 20 seconds or until browned.

**3.** Arrange 1 sliced tomato on each bread slice. Sprinkle ⅛ teaspoon oregano and basil over each bread slice. Top with zucchini and shallot. Arrange sliced olives over vegetables. Sprinkle 1½ tablespoons cheese on each serving.

**4.** Place bruschetta on grill rack or vegetable grate 2 minutes or until cheese is melted and bruschetta is hot. Or place on baking sheet and broil 20 to 30 seconds until cheese melts.

**MAKES 2 SERVINGS**

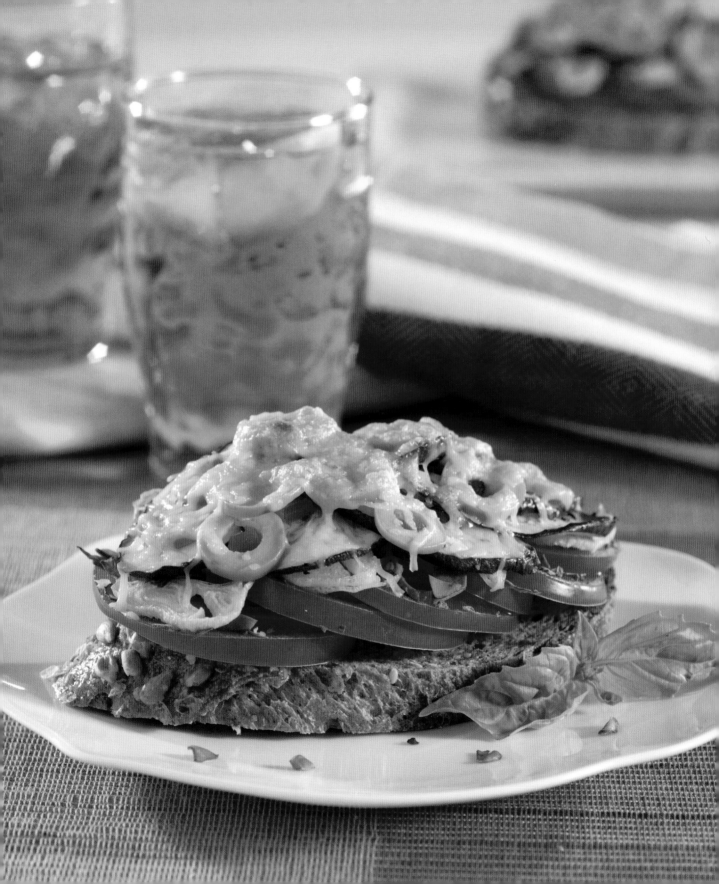

# FARRO VEGGIE BURGERS

1½ cups water*

½ cup pearled farro or spelt*

2 medium potatoes, peeled and quartered

2 to 4 tablespoons canola oil, divided

¾ cup finely chopped green onions

1 cup grated carrots

2 teaspoons grated fresh ginger

2 tablespoons ground almonds

¼ to ¾ teaspoon salt

¼ teaspoon black pepper

½ cup panko bread crumbs

6 whole wheat hamburger buns

Ketchup and mustard (optional)

*Use 2 cups water if using spelt.

**1.** Combine 1½ cups water and farro in medium saucepan; bring to a boil over high heat. Reduce heat to low; partially cover and cook 25 to 30 minutes or until farro is tender. Drain and cool. (If using spelt, use 2 cups of water and cook until tender.)

**2.** Meanwhile, place potatoes in large saucepan; cover with water. Bring to a boil; reduce heat and simmer 20 minutes or until tender. Cool and mash potatoes; set aside.

**3.** Heat 1 tablespoon oil in medium skillet over medium-high heat. Add green onions; cook and stir 1 minute. Add carrots and ginger; cover and cook 2 to 3 minutes or until carrots are tender. Transfer to large bowl; cool completely.

**4.** Add mashed potatoes and farro to carrot mixture. Add almonds, salt and pepper; mix well. Shape mixture into six patties. Spread panko on medium plate; coat patties with panko.

**5.** Heat 1 tablespoon oil in large nonstick skillet over medium heat. Cook patties about 4 minutes per side or until golden brown, adding additional oil as needed. Serve on buns with desired condiments.

**MAKES 6 SERVINGS**

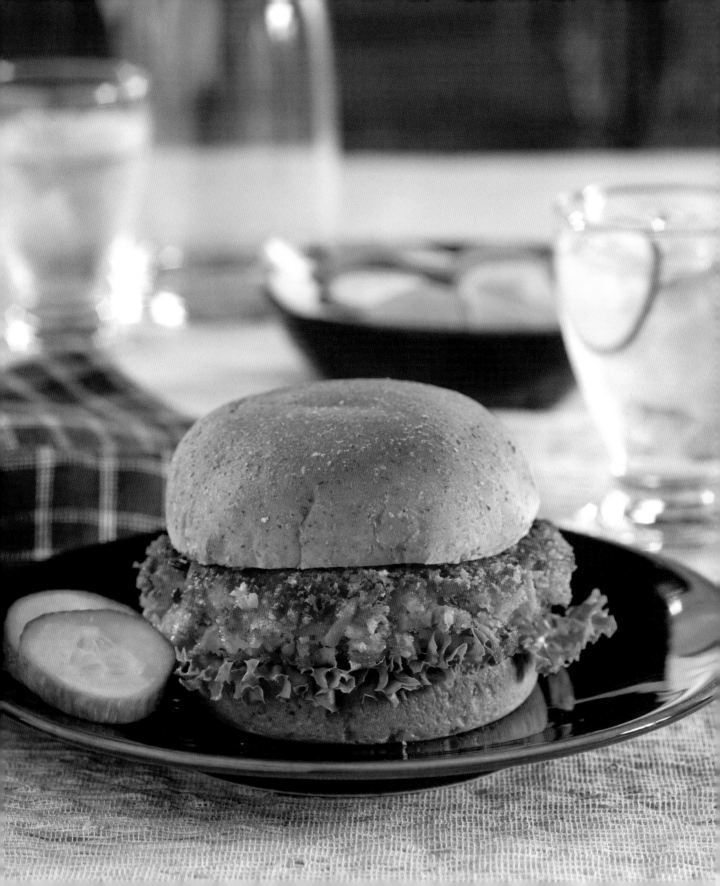

# MEDITERRANEAN ROASTED VEGETABLE WRAPS

1 **head cauliflower, cut into 1-inch florets**

4 **tablespoons olive oil, divided**

2 **teaspoons ras el hanout, 7-spice blend, shawarma blend or za'atar**

1 **teaspoon salt, divided**

1 **zucchini, quartered lengthwise and cut into ¼-inch pieces**

1 **yellow squash, quartered lengthwise and cut into ¼-inch pieces**

½ **red onion, thinly sliced**

¼ **cup red pepper sauce (avjar)**

4 **large thin pitas or lavash (10 inches)**

4 **ounces feta cheese, crumbled**

1 **cup cooked chickpeas**

¼ **cup diced tomatoes**

¼ **cup minced fresh parsley**

¼ **cup diced cucumber (optional)**

2 **teaspoons vegetable oil**

**1.** Preheat oven to 400°F. Combine cauliflower, 2 tablespoons olive oil, ras el hanout and ½ teaspoon salt in large bowl; toss to coat. Spread on half of sheet pan. Combine zucchini, yellow squash, onion, remaining 2 tablespoons olive oil and ½ teaspoon salt in same bowl; toss to coat. Spread on other side of sheet pan. Roast 25 minutes or until vegetables are browned and tender, stirring once. Remove from oven; cool slightly.

**2.** Spread 1 tablespoon red pepper sauce on one pita. Top with one fourth of vegetables, feta, chickpeas, tomatoes, parsley and cucumber, if desired. Fold two sides over filling; roll up into burrito shape. Repeat with remaining ingredients.

**3.** Heat 1 teaspoon vegetable oil in large skillet over medium-high heat. Add two wraps, seam sides down; cook 1 minute or until browned. Turn and cook other side until browned. Repeat with remaining vegetable oil and wraps. Cut in half to serve.

**MAKES 4 SERVINGS**

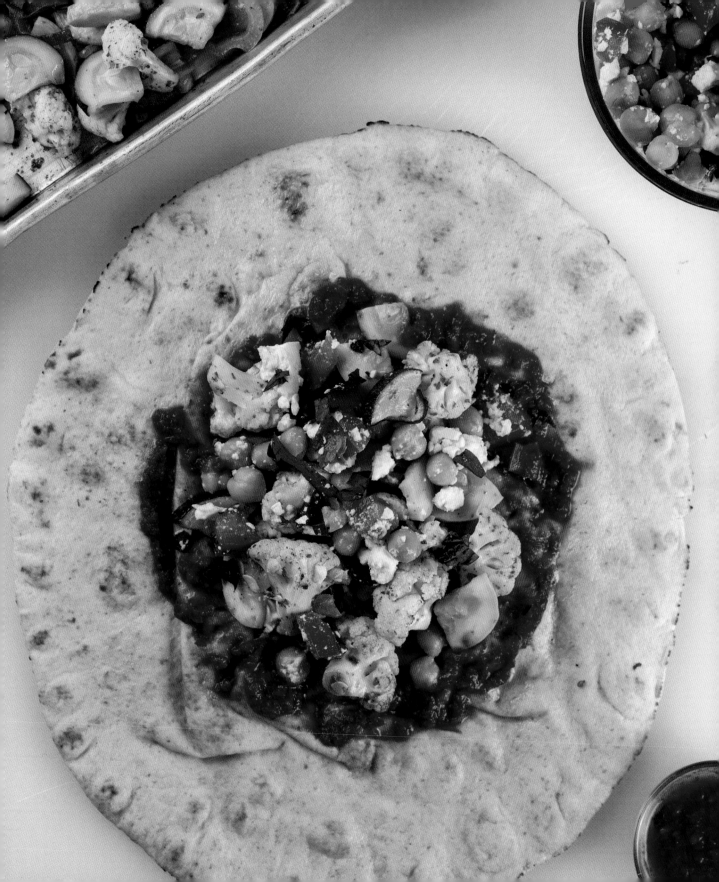

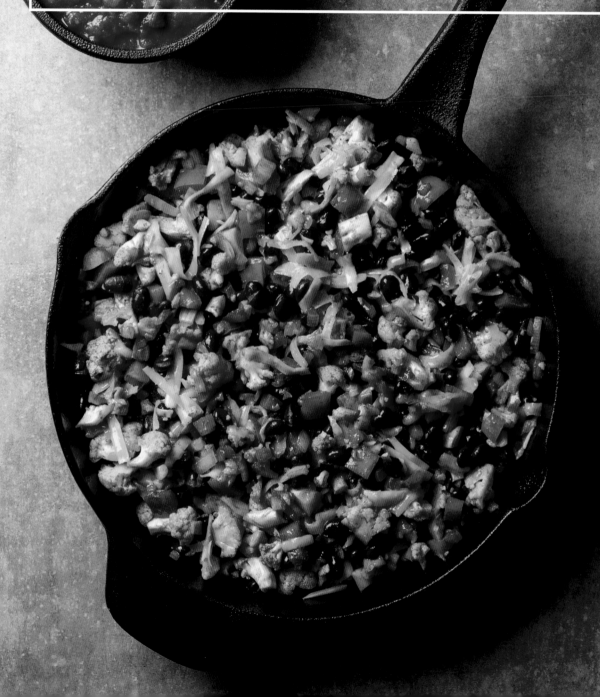

# CHAPTER 4

# MAIN DISHES

# MEXICAN CAULIFLOWER AND BEAN SKILLET

1 teaspoon olive oil

3 cups coarsely chopped cauliflower

¾ teaspoon salt

½ medium yellow onion, chopped

1 green bell pepper, chopped

1 clove garlic, minced

1 teaspoon chili powder

¾ teaspoon ground cumin

Dash of ground red pepper

1 can (15 ounces) black beans, rinsed and drained

1 cup (4 ounces) shredded Cheddar-Jack cheese

Salsa and sour cream

**1.** Heat oil in large cast iron skillet over medium-high heat. Add cauliflower and salt; cook and stir 5 minutes. Add onion, bell pepper, garlic, chili powder, cumin and ground red pepper; cook and stir 5 minutes or until cauliflower is tender. Add beans; cook until beans are heated through. Remove from heat.

**2.** Sprinkle with cheese; fold gently and let stand until melted. Serve with salsa and sour cream.

**MAKES 4 TO 6 SERVINGS**

# FRIED GREEN TOMATO PARMESAN

2 cans (15 ounces each) tomato sauce

4 green tomatoes, thickly sliced into 3 slices each

½ teaspoon salt, divided

Black pepper

½ cup all-purpose flour

1 teaspoon Italian seasoning

2 eggs

2 tablespoons water

1½ cups panko bread crumbs

4 tablespoons olive oil

½ cup shredded Parmesan cheese

Shredded fresh basil

Hot cooked spaghetti

**1.** Preheat oven to 350°F. Spread 1 cup tomato sauce in 9-inch square baking dish. Sprinkle one side of tomatoes with ¼ teaspoon salt; season lightly with pepper.

**2.** Combine flour, Italian seasoning and remaining ¼ teaspoon salt in shallow bowl. Whisk eggs and water in another shallow bowl. Place panko in third shallow bowl. Coat tomatoes with flour mixture. Dip in egg mixture. Dredge in panko, pressing onto all sides.

**3.** Heat 2 tablespoons oil in large skillet over medium-high heat. Add half of tomatoes; cook 3 minutes per side or until panko is golden brown. Arrange tomatoes in single layer in sauce in baking dish. Sprinkle 1 teaspoon cheese on each tomato; spread some sauce over tomatoes. Heat remaining 2 tablespoons oil in same skillet; cook remaining tomatoes 3 minutes per side until coating is golden brown. Stagger tomatoes in second layer over tomatoes in baking dish. Top each tomato with 1 teaspoon cheese and spread 1 cup sauce over top. Sprinkle with remaining cheese.

**4.** Bake 20 minutes or until cheese is melted and sauce is heated through. Heat remaining tomato sauce. Serve tomatoes with basil, spaghetti and sauce.

**MAKES 4 SERVINGS**

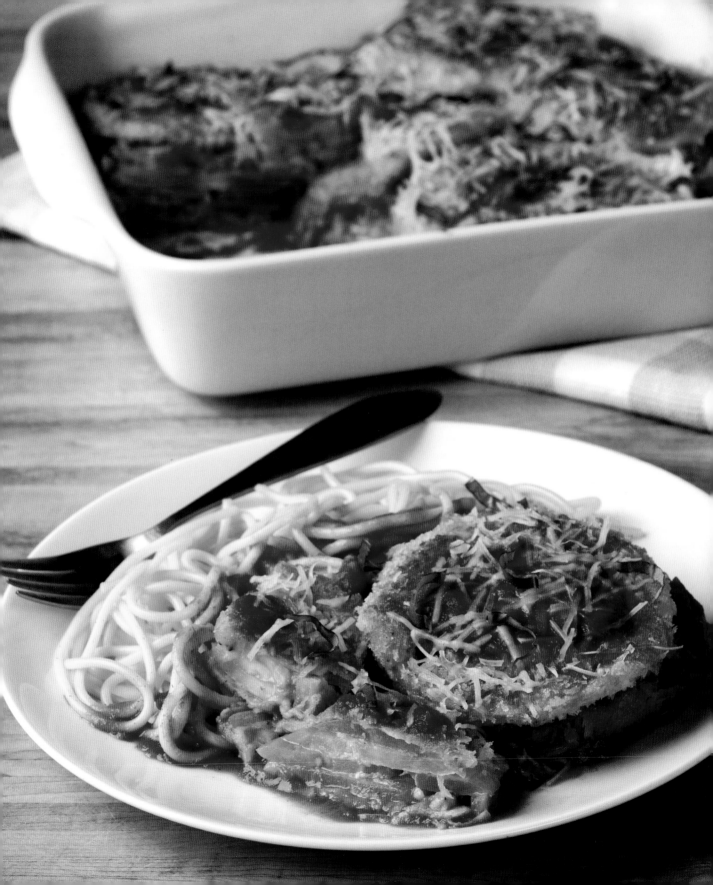

# TACO SALAD SUPREME

## CHILI

- **1 pound refrigerated plant-based ground meatless product** *or* **1 package (10 ounces) frozen meatless crumbles**
- **1 medium onion, chopped**
- **1 stalk celery, chopped**
- **2 medium fresh tomatoes, chopped**
- **1 jalapeño pepper, finely chopped**
- **1½ teaspoons chili powder**
- **1 teaspoon salt**
- **1 teaspoon ground cumin**
- **½ teaspoon black pepper**
- **1 can (15 ounces) tomato sauce**
- **1 can (about 15 ounces) kidney beans, rinsed and drained**
- **1 can (about 15 ounces) pinto beans, rinsed and drained**
- **1 cup water**

## SALAD

- **8 cups chopped romaine lettuce (large pieces)**
- **2 cups diced fresh tomatoes**
- **48 small round tortilla chips**
- **1 cup salsa**
- **½ cup sour cream**
- **1 cup (4 ounces) shredded Cheddar cheese**

**1.** Combine meatless product, onion and celery in large saucepan; cook over medium-high heat 6 to 8 minutes or until meatless product is browned, stirring to break into crumbles.

**2.** Add chopped tomatoes, jalapeño, chili powder, salt, cumin and black pepper; cook and stir 1 minute. Stir in tomato sauce, beans and water; bring to a boil. Reduce heat to medium-low; cook about 30 minutes or until most of liquid is absorbed.

**3.** For each salad, combine 2 cups lettuce and ½ cup diced tomatoes in individual bowl. Top with 12 tortilla chips, ¾ cup chili, ¼ cup salsa and 2 tablespoons sour cream. Sprinkle with ¼ cup cheese. (Reserve remaining chili for another use.)

**MAKES 4 SERVINGS**

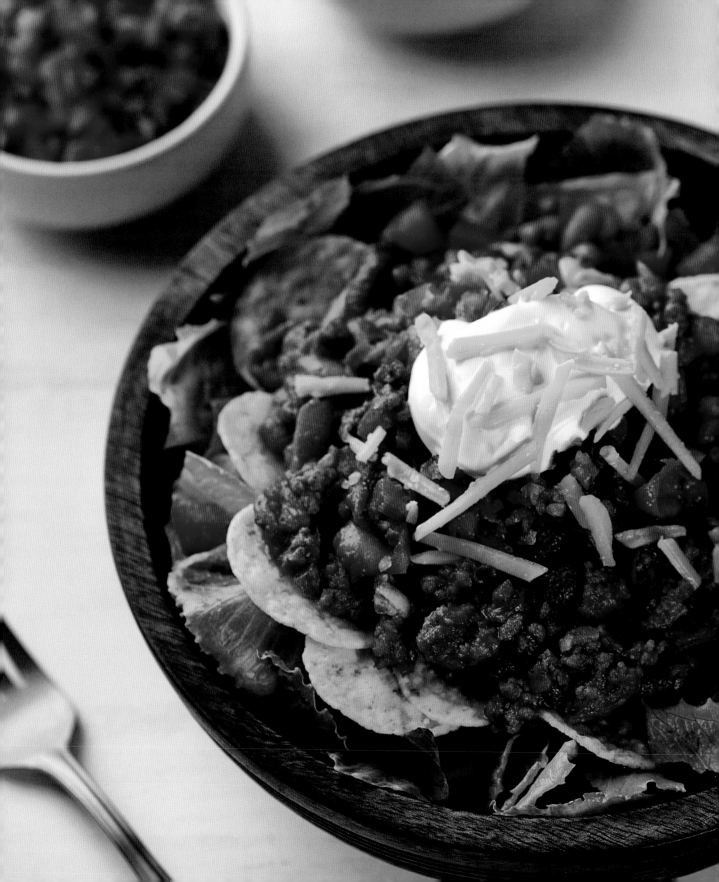

# LEEK AND CHIVE CHAMP

3 medium russet
   potatoes
   (1½ pounds), peeled
   and cut into 1-inch
   pieces

6 tablespoons (¾ stick)
   butter, divided

2 large leeks, halved and
   sliced

½ cup milk

¼ cup chopped fresh
   chives

½ teaspoon salt

¼ teaspoon black pepper

½ cup prepared French
   fried onions
   (optional)

**1.** Place potatoes in large saucepan; add cold water to cover by 2 inches. Bring to a boil over medium-high heat; cook 16 to 18 minutes or until tender. Drain and return to saucepan.

**2.** Meanwhile, melt 2 tablespoons butter in medium skillet over medium heat. Add leeks; cook 5 to 6 minutes or until tender, stirring occasionally.

**3.** Heat milk in small saucepan over medium-high heat until hot. Add 2 tablespoons butter; cook until melted. Pour milk mixture into saucepan with potatoes; mash until smooth. Stir in leeks, chives, salt and pepper; mix well.

**4.** Spoon into serving bowl; make large indentation in top of potatoes. Melt remaining 2 tablespoons butter; pour into indentation. Sprinkle with fried onions, if desired.

**MAKES 4 TO 6 SERVINGS**

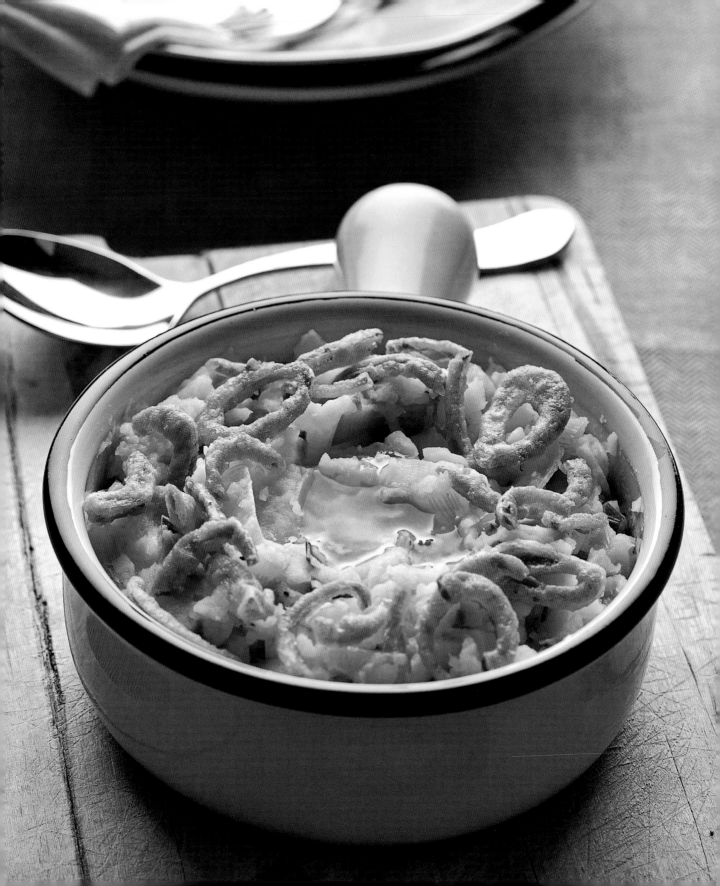

# CORNMEAL-CRUSTED CAULIFLOWER STEAKS

½ cup cornmeal

¼ cup all-purpose flour

1 teaspoon salt

1 teaspoon dried sage

½ teaspoon garlic powder

Black pepper

½ cup milk

2 heads cauliflower

4 tablespoons butter, melted

Coleslaw and barbecue sauce (optional)

**1.** Preheat oven to 400°F. Line baking sheet with parchment paper.

**2.** Combine cornmeal, flour, salt, sage and garlic powder in shallow bowl or baking pan. Season with pepper. Pour milk into another shallow bowl.

**3.** Turn cauliflower stem side up on cutting board. Trim away leaves, leaving stem intact. Slice through stem into 2 or 3 slices. Trim off excess florets from two end slices, creating flat "steaks." Repeat with remaining cauliflower; reserve extra cauliflower for another use.

**4.** Dip cauliflower into milk to coat both sides. Place in cornmeal mixture; pat onto all sides of cauliflower. Place on prepared baking sheet. Drizzle butter evenly over cauliflower.

**5.** Bake 40 minutes or until cauliflower is tender. Serve with coleslaw on the side and barbecue sauce for dipping, if desired.

**MAKES 4 SERVINGS**

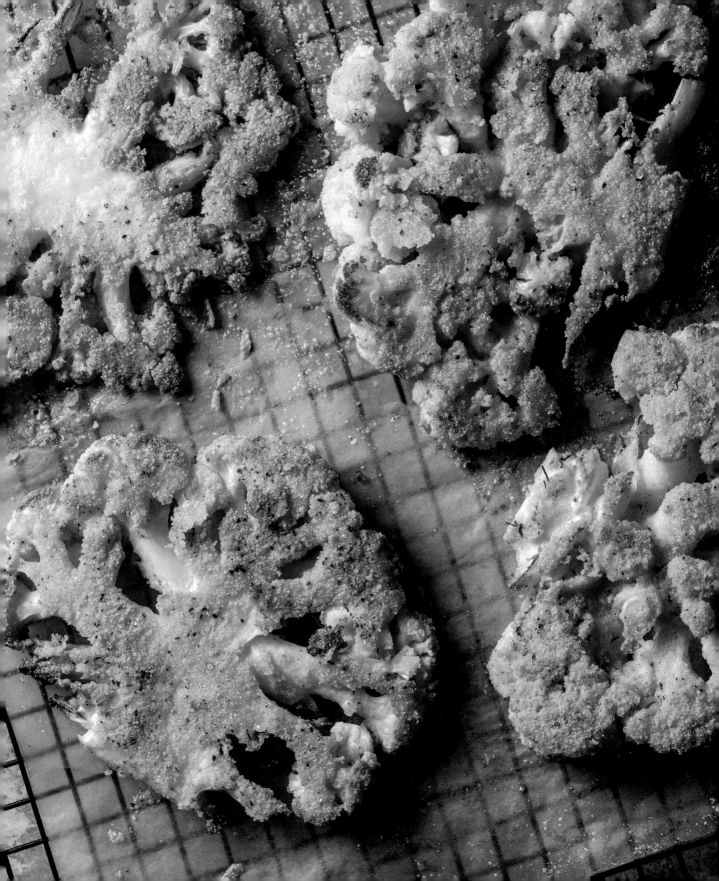

# SESAME NOODLE BOWL

1 package (16 ounces) uncooked spaghetti

6 tablespoons soy sauce

5 tablespoons dark sesame oil

3 tablespoons sugar

3 tablespoons rice vinegar

4 tablespoons vegetable oil, divided

3 cloves garlic, minced

1 teaspoon grated fresh ginger or ginger paste

½ teaspoon sriracha sauce

2 green onions, sliced

1 red bell pepper

1 cucumber

1 carrot

1 package (14 to 16 ounces) firm tofu, drained and patted dry

Sesame seeds (optional)

**1.** Cook spaghetti according to package directions until al dente in large saucepan of boiling salted water. Drain, reserving 1 tablespoon water.

**2.** Whisk soy sauce, sesame oil, sugar, vinegar, 2 tablespoons vegetable oil, garlic, ginger and sriracha in large bowl. Stir in noodles, reserved pasta cooking water and green onions. Let stand at least 30 minutes until noodles have cooled to room temperature and most of sauce is absorbed, stirring occasionally.

**3.** Meanwhile, cut bell pepper into thin strips. Peel cucumber and carrot and shred with julienne peeler into long strands, or cut into thin strips.

**4.** Cut tofu into thin triangles or 1-inch cubes. Heat remaining 2 tablespoons vegetable oil in large nonstick skillet over high heat. Add tofu; cook 5 minutes or until browned on both sides, turning occasionally.

**5.** Place noodles in bowls. Top with tofu, bell pepper, cucumber and carrot. Sprinkle with sesame seeds, if desired.

**MAKES 6 SERVINGS**

TIP

Sesame noodles are great served warm or cold. To serve them cold, cover and refrigerate a few hours or overnight after step 2 before preparing the vegetables and tofu. For a side dish or potluck dish, skip the tofu and stir the vegetables into the noodles after they are cool. Refrigerate until ready to serve.

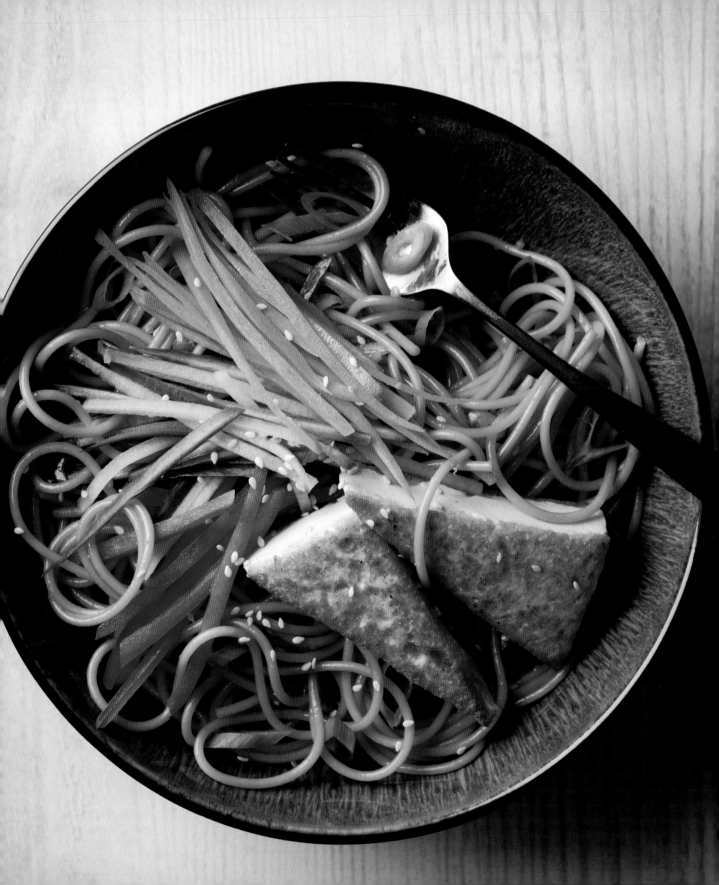

# VEGETARIAN LASAGNA

1 tablespoon olive oil

1 pound refrigerated
   plant-based ground
   meatless product

1 medium onion,
   chopped

3 cloves garlic, minced,
   divided

1½ teaspoons salt, divided

1 can (28 ounces)
   crushed tomatoes

1 can (28 ounces) diced
   tomatoes

2 teaspoons Italian
   seasoning

1 egg

1 container (15 ounces)
   ricotta cheese

¾ cup grated Parmesan
   cheese, divided

½ cup minced fresh
   parsley

¼ teaspoon black pepper

12 uncooked no-boil
   lasagna noodles

4 cups (16 ounces)
   shredded mozzarella

**1.** Preheat oven to 350°F. Spray 13×9-inch baking dish with nonstick cooking spray.

**2.** Heat oil in large saucepan over medium-high heat. Add meatless product, onion, 2 cloves garlic and 1 teaspoon salt; cook and stir 10 minutes or until meatless product is browned, breaking into crumbles. Add crushed tomatoes, diced tomatoes and Italian seasoning; bring to a boil. Reduce heat to medium-low; cook 15 minutes, stirring occasionally.

**3.** Meanwhile, beat egg in medium bowl. Stir in ricotta, ½ cup Parmesan, parsley, remaining 1 clove garlic, ½ teaspoon salt and pepper until well blended.

**4.** Spread ¼ cup sauce in prepared baking dish. Top with 3 noodles, breaking to fit if necessary. Spread one third of ricotta mixture over noodles. Sprinkle with 1 cup mozzarella; top with 2 cups sauce. Repeat layers of noodles, ricotta mixture, mozzarella and sauce two times. Top with remaining 3 noodles, sauce, 1 cup mozzarella and ¼ cup Parmesan. Cover dish with foil sprayed with cooking spray.

**5.** Bake 30 minutes. Remove foil; bake 20 minutes or until hot and bubbly and cheese is lightly browned. Let stand 10 minutes before serving.

**MAKES 6 TO 8 SERVINGS**

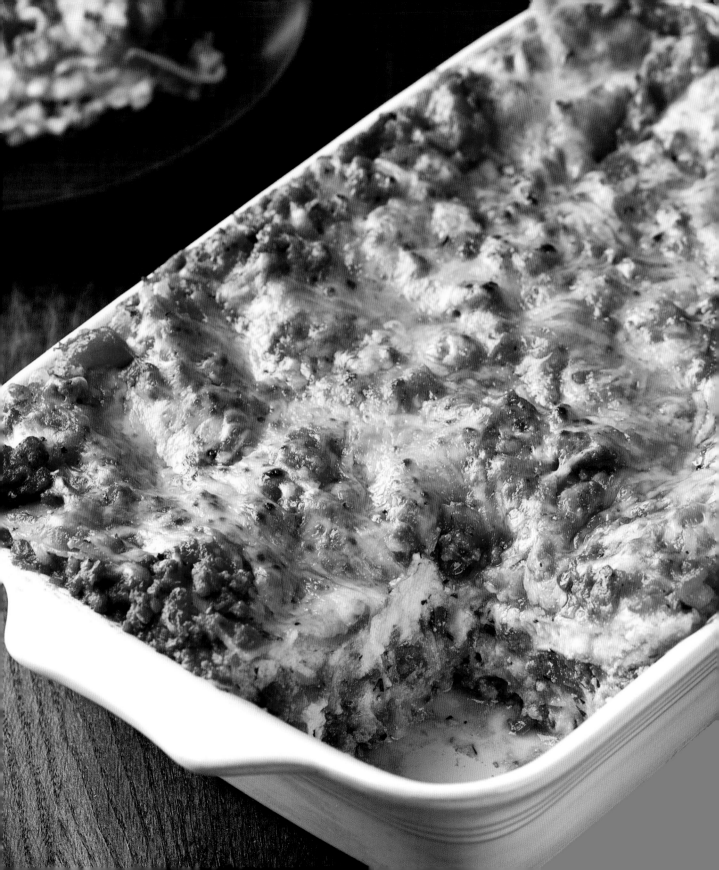

# SOBA TERIYAKI BOWL

¾ **cup plus 1 tablespoon cornstarch, divided**

2 **teaspoons salt, divided**

½ **cup plus 2 tablespoons water, divided**

1 **head cauliflower, cut into 1-inch florets**

¾ **cup pineapple juice**

¾ **cup soy sauce**

2 **tablespoons packed brown sugar**

1 **tablespoon lime juice**

1 **teaspoon minced garlic**

6 **ounces uncooked soba noodles**

5 **cups shredded red, green or mixed cabbage *or* 1 package (14 ounces) coleslaw mix**

½ **cup unseasoned rice vinegar**

1 **teaspoon granulated sugar**

2 **green onions, chopped**

1 **tablespoon sesame seeds**

**1.** Preheat oven to 400°F. Spray sheet pan with nonstick cooking spray. Whisk ¾ cup cornstarch and 1 teaspoon salt in medium bowl. Whisk in ½ cup water until smooth. Dip cauliflower into mixture; place in single layer on prepared sheet pan. Bake 20 minutes or until tender.

**2.** Meanwhile, bring pineapple juice, soy sauce, brown sugar, lime juice and garlic to a simmer in small saucepan. Whisk remaining 2 tablespoons water into remaining 1 tablespoon cornstarch in small bowl; stir into sauce. Reduce heat to low; cook and stir 5 minutes. Transfer to large bowl; cool slightly. Remove ¼ cup sauce; set aside.

**3.** Cook soba noodles according to package directions. Drain and rinse under cold water until cool. Divide among serving bowls.

**4.** Combine cabbage, vinegar, granulated sugar and remaining 1 teaspoon salt in medium bowl; mix and squeeze with hands until well blended.

**5.** Add cauliflower to large bowl of sauce; stir to coat. Divide among serving bowls. Drizzle some of reserved sauce over noodles. Serve with cabbage mixture. Sprinkle with green onions and sesame seeds.

**MAKES 4 SERVINGS**

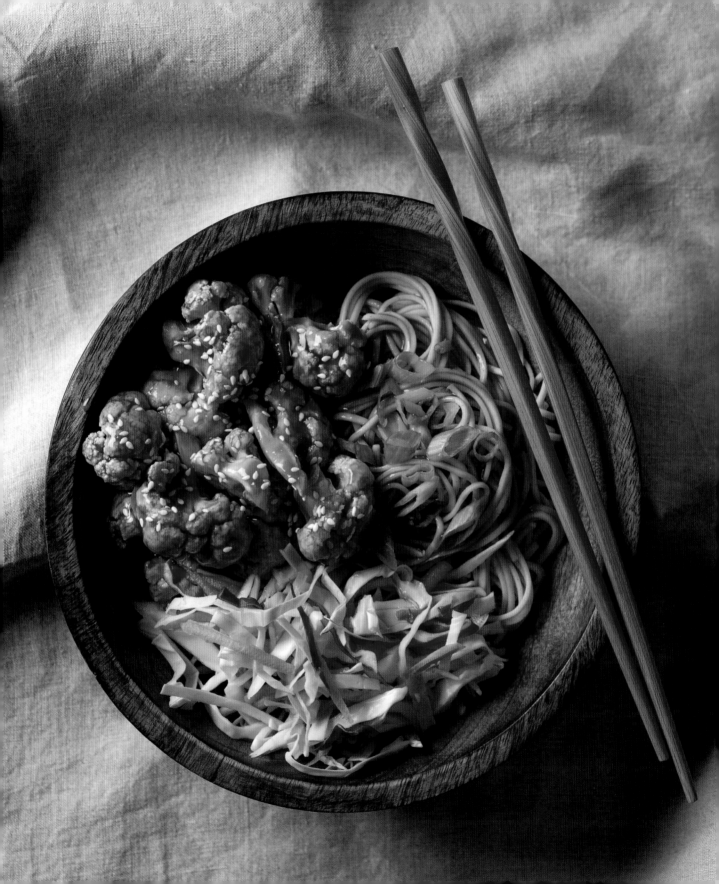

# LENTIL BOLOGNESE

2  tablespoons olive oil

1  onion, chopped

1  carrot, chopped

1  stalk celery, chopped

2  cloves garlic, minced

1  teaspoon salt

½  teaspoon dried
   oregano

   Pinch red pepper flakes

3  tablespoons tomato
   paste

¼  cup dry white wine

1  can (28 ounces)
   crushed tomatoes

1  can (about 14 ounces)
   diced tomatoes

1  cup dried lentils, rinsed

1  portobello mushroom,
   gills removed, finely
   chopped

1½ cups water or
   vegetable broth

   Hot cooked pasta

**1.** Heat oil in large saucepan over medium heat. Add onion, carrot and celery; cook and stir 10 minutes or until onion is lightly browned and carrot is softened.

**2.** Stir in garlic, salt, oregano and red pepper flakes. Add tomato paste; cook and stir 1 minute. Add wine; cook and stir until absorbed. Stir in crushed tomatoes, diced tomatoes, lentils, mushroom and water. Bring to a simmer.

**3.** Reduce heat to medium; partially cover and simmer about 40 minutes or until lentils are tender, removing cover after 20 minutes. Serve over pasta.

**MAKES 6 TO 8 SERVINGS**

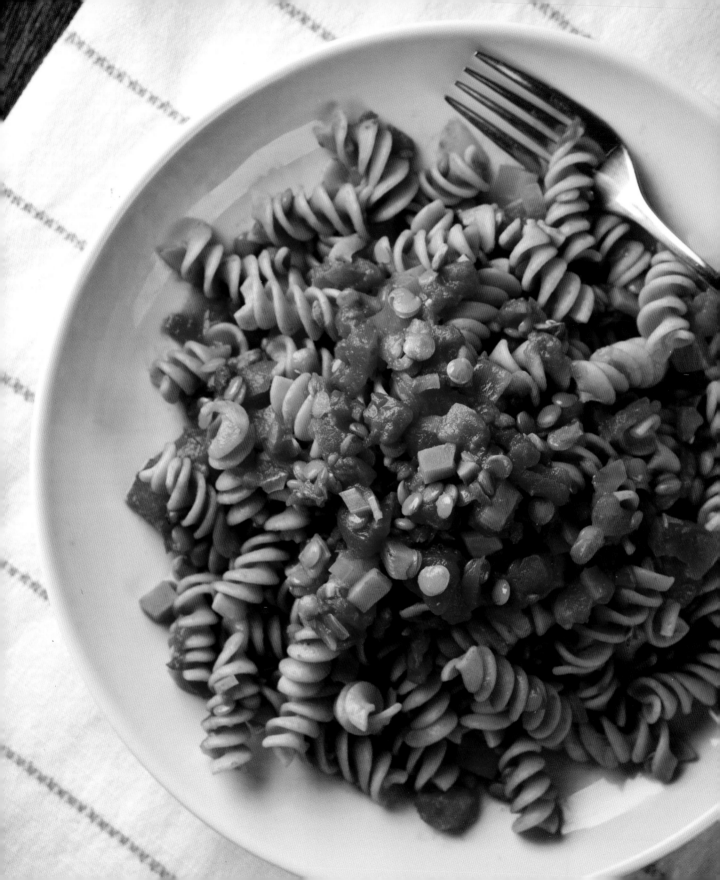

# LEMON CREAM PASTA WITH ROASTED CAULIFLOWER

1 head cauliflower
(2½ pounds), cut into
1-inch florets

2 tablespoons olive oil

1 teaspoon salt, divided

¼ teaspoon plus
⅛ teaspoon black
pepper, divided

8 ounces uncooked
cavatappi pasta

¼ cup (½ stick) butter, cut
into pieces

¼ cup all-purpose flour

2 cups milk

½ cup shredded
Parmesan cheese

Grated peel and juice
of 1 lemon

¼ cup chopped almonds,
toasted

Baby arugula

Aleppo pepper or
red pepper flakes
(optional)

**1.** Preheat oven to 425°F. Place cauliflower on sheet pan. Drizzle with oil and sprinkle with ½ teaspoon salt and ¼ teaspoon black pepper; toss to coat. Roast 35 to 45 minutes or until cauliflower is well browned and tender.

**2.** Cook pasta in large saucepan of boiling salted water according to package directions until al dente. Drain, reserving 1 cup pasta cooking water. Place pasta in large bowl; add cauliflower.

**3.** Melt butter in same saucepan over medium heat; whisk in flour until smooth paste forms. Whisk in milk, remaining ½ teaspoon salt and ⅛ teaspoon black pepper; cook 2 to 3 minutes or until thickened. Whisk in ½ cup reserved pasta water and Parmesan until smooth. Pour over pasta and cauliflower; stir to coat. Add additional pasta water by tablespoonfuls to loosen sauce, if needed. Stir in lemon juice and almonds. Top with arugula or gently fold into pasta mixture. Sprinkle with lemon peel and Aleppo pepper.

**MAKES 6 TO 8 SERVINGS**

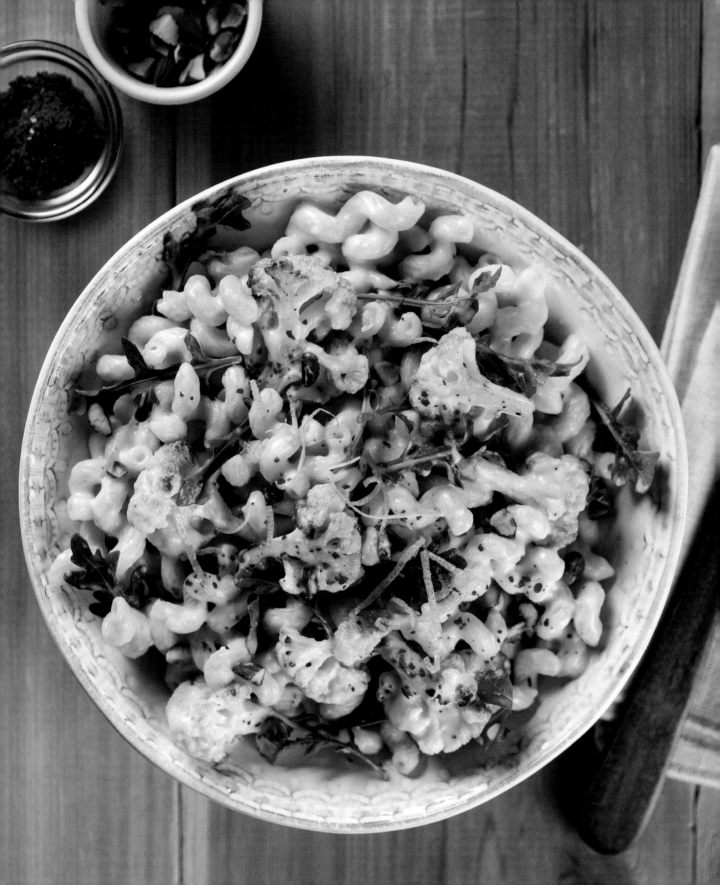

# PEANUT BUTTER TOFU BOWL

## SAUCE

- ¼ cup peanut butter
- ¼ cup hoisin sauce
- 1 tablespoon packed brown sugar
- 1 tablespoon dark sesame oil
- 1 tablespoon water
- 1½ teaspoons minced fresh ginger
- 1½ teaspoons unseasoned rice vinegar
- 1½ teaspoons soy sauce
- 1 clove garlic, minced
- ½ teaspoon sriracha sauce

## BOWL

- 1 package (14 to 16 ounces) firm tofu, cut into 24 (1-inch) cubes
- ¼ cup cornstarch
- 2 tablespoons plus 1 teaspoon vegetable oil, divided
- 1 head bok choy
- 1 clove garlic, minced
- 1 tablespoon soy sauce
- 1 tablespoon rice vinegar
- 2 cups hot cooked rice
- Minced fresh cilantro and/or chopped peanuts (optional)

**1.** For sauce, combine peanut butter, hoisin, brown sugar, sesame oil, 1 tablespoon water, ginger, 1½ teaspoons vinegar, 1½ teaspoons soy sauce, 1 clove garlic and sriracha in small saucepan. Cook over medium-low heat 5 minutes, whisking frequently.

**2.** Toss tofu with cornstarch in large bowl. Heat 2 tablespoons vegetable oil in large nonstick skillet over high heat. Add tofu to skillet; cook without stirring 5 minutes or until well browned and crusted on bottom. Turn and cook 5 minutes or until browned on other side. Cook 2 minutes, turning frequently until other sides of tofu are lightly browned. Add sauce; cook 1 minute or until tofu is glazed.

**3.** Meanwhile, separate leaves and stems of bok choy. Coarsely chop stems and leaves separately. Heat remaining 1 teaspoon vegetable oil in medium skillet over medium-high heat. Add bok choy stems; cook and stir 3 minutes. Add leaves and 1 clove garlic; cook and stir 1 minute. Add 1 tablespoon soy sauce and 1 tablespoon vinegar; cook and stir 30 seconds.

**4.** Divide tofu, bok choy and rice among bowls. Garnish with cilantro and peanuts.

**MAKES 4 SERVINGS**

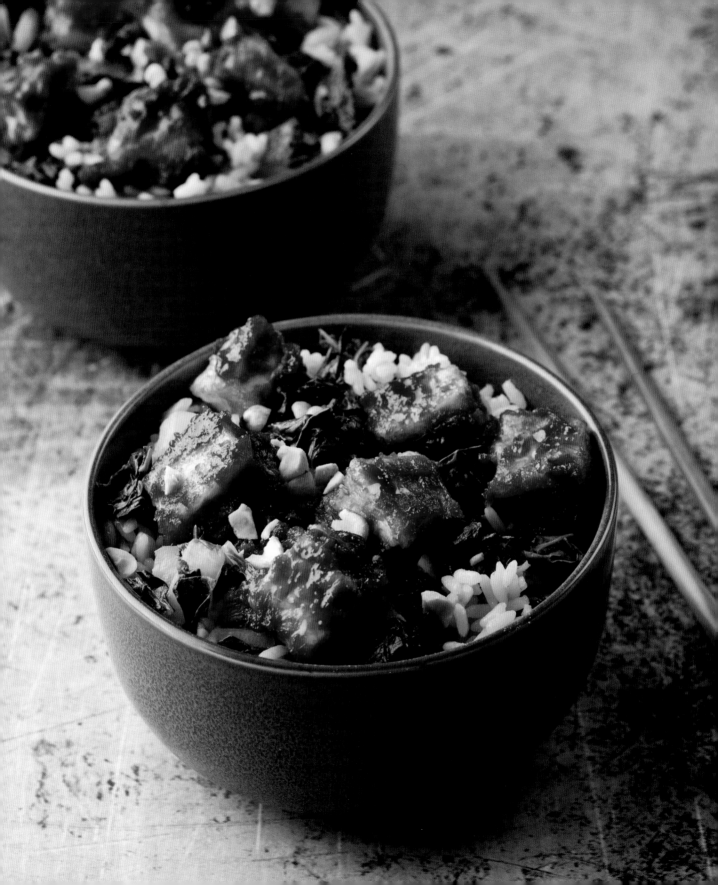

# RED BEANS AND RICE WITH PICKLED CARROTS AND CUCUMBERS

1 **pound dried red kidney beans**

1 **tablespoon plus 1 teaspoon salt, divided**

**Pickled Carrots and Cucumbers (page 109)**

2 **tablespoons olive oil**

2 **onions, chopped**

3 **stalks celery, chopped**

1 **green bell pepper, chopped**

4 **cloves garlic, minced**

4 **cups vegetable broth**

1 **teaspoon liquid smoke**

1 **bay leaf**

2 **teaspoons Italian seasoning**

½ **teaspoon black pepper**

¼ **teaspoon ground red pepper**

**Hot cooked brown rice**

**Sliced avocado**

**Hot pepper sauce**

**1.** Place beans in large bowl. Cover with water and stir in 1 tablespoon salt. Soak 8 hours or overnight. Meanwhile, prepare pickled carrots and cucumbers.

**2.** Heat oil in large saucepan over medium-high heat. Add onions; cook and stir 5 minutes. Stir in 1 teaspoon salt. Add celery, bell pepper and garlic; cook and stir 5 minutes or until vegetables are tender.

**3.** Drain beans; add to saucepan with broth, liquid smoke, bay leaf, Italian seasoning, black pepper and red pepper. Bring to a boil. Reduce heat; simmer, partially covered, 45 minutes.

**4.** Remove 2 cups bean mixture to medium bowl; let stand 15 minutes to cool slightly. Place in blender or food processor and add ½ cup water; blend until smooth. Stir into beans; continue to cook until beans are tender. Taste and season with additional salt, if desired. Serve with rice, pickled carrots and cucumbers, avocado and hot pepper sauce.

**MAKES 6 SERVINGS**

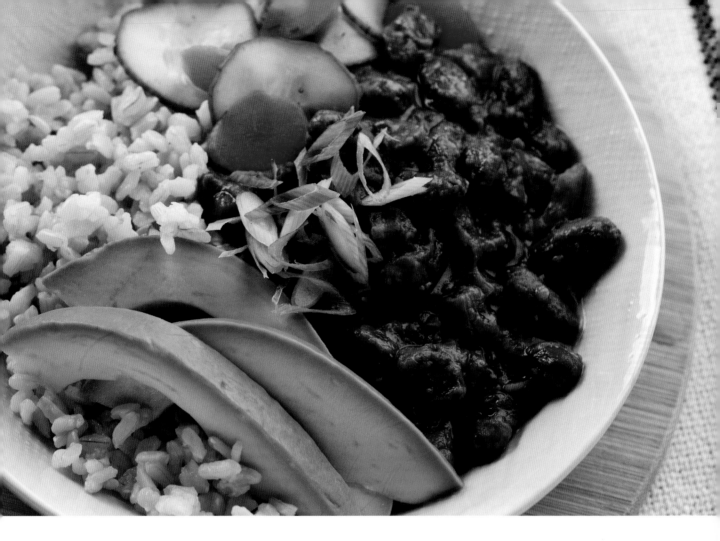

# PICKLED CARROTS AND CUCUMBERS

2  carrots, peeled

1  cucumber

¼  cup water

2  tablespoons sugar

1  tablespoon salt

1  teaspoon peppercorns

2  cloves garlic, smashed

¼  teaspoon dried dill

2  bay leaves

1½  cups white vinegar

**1.** Thinly slice carrots into coins. Very thinly slice cucumber (¹⁄₁₆-inch slices) with a mandoline if you have one. Place carrots and cucumbers in 1-quart jar.

**2.** Combine water, sugar, salt, peppercorns, garlic, dill and bay leaves in small saucepan. Cook over medium heat just until salt and sugar are dissolved. Pour over vegetables in jar. Add enough vinegar to cover. Seal jar and refrigerate at least 2 hours. Can be made a few days in advance.

# CHICKPEA TIKKA MASALA

- **1 tablespoon olive oil**
- **1 onion, chopped**
- **3 cloves garlic, minced**
- **1 tablespoon minced fresh ginger or ginger paste**
- **1 tablespoon garam masala**
- **1 teaspoon ground cumin**
- **1 teaspoon ground coriander**
- **1 teaspoon salt**
- **¼ teaspoon ground red pepper**
- **2 cans (15 ounces each) chickpeas, drained**
- **1 can (28 ounces) crushed tomatoes**
- **1 can (about 13 ounces) coconut milk**
- **1 package (about 12 ounces) firm silken tofu, drained and cut into 1-inch cubes**
- **Hot cooked brown basmati rice**
- **Chopped fresh cilantro**

**1.** Heat oil in large saucepan over medium-high heat. Add onion; cook and stir 5 minutes or until translucent. Add garlic, ginger, garam masala, cumin, coriander, salt and red pepper; cook and stir 1 minute.

**2.** Stir in chickpeas, tomatoes and coconut milk; simmer 30 minutes or until thickened and chickpeas have softened slightly. Add tofu; stir gently. Cook 7 to 10 minutes or until tofu is heated through. Serve over rice; garnish with cilantro.

**MAKES 4 SERVINGS**

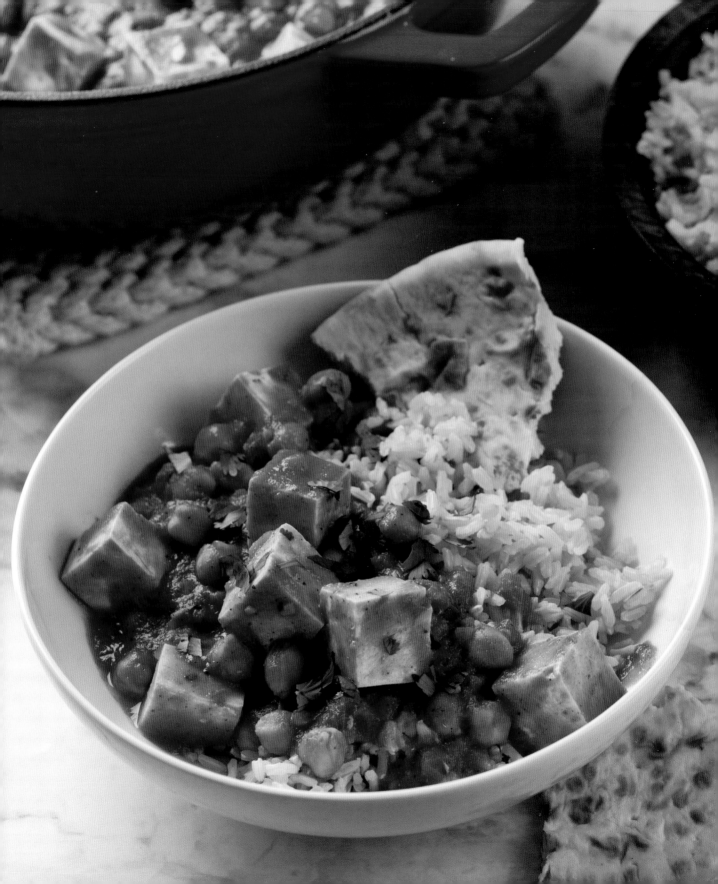

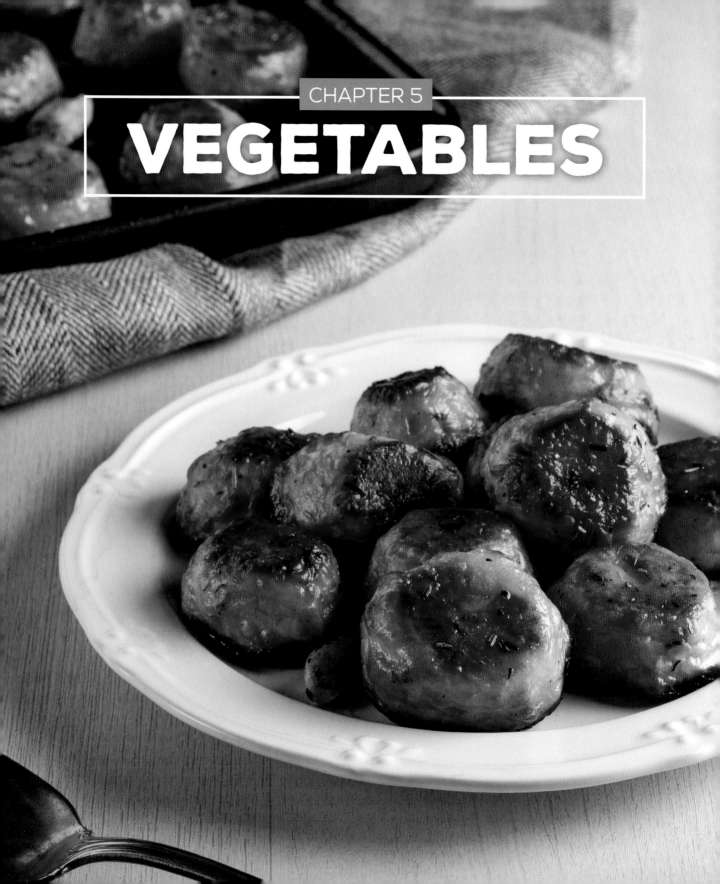

# CHAPTER 5

# VEGETABLES

# CREAMY SLAB POTATOES

¼ cup (½ stick) butter, melted

1 teaspoon salt

½ teaspoon dried rosemary

½ teaspoon dried thyme

¼ teaspoon black pepper

2½ pounds Yukon Gold potatoes, peeled and cut crosswise into 1-inch slices (6 to 8 potatoes)

1 cup water

3 cloves garlic, smashed

1. Preheat oven to 500°F.

2. Combine butter, salt, rosemary, thyme and pepper in 13×9-inch baking pan (do not use glass); mix well. Add potatoes; toss to coat. Spread in single layer.

3. Bake 15 minutes. Turn potatoes; bake 15 minutes. Add water and garlic to pan; bake 15 minutes. Remove to serving plate; pour any remaining liquid in pan over potatoes.

**MAKES 4 SERVINGS**

# CREAMED SPINACH

1 **pound baby spinach**

½ **cup (1 stick) butter**

2 **tablespoons finely chopped onion**

¼ **cup all-purpose flour**

2 **cups whole milk**

1 **bay leaf**

½ **teaspoon salt**

**Pinch ground nutmeg**

**Pinch ground red pepper**

**Black pepper**

**1.** Bring medium saucepan of water to a boil over high heat. Add spinach; cook 1 minute. Drain and transfer to bowl of ice water to stop cooking. Squeeze spinach dry; coarsely chop. Wipe out saucepan with paper towel.

**2.** Melt butter in same saucepan over medium heat. Add onion; cook and stir 2 minutes or until softened. Add flour; cook and stir 2 to 3 minutes or until slightly golden. Slowly add milk in thin, steady stream, whisking constantly until mixture boils and begins to thicken. Stir in bay leaf, ½ teaspoon salt, nutmeg and red pepper. Reduce heat to low; cook 5 minutes, stirring frequently. Remove and discard bay leaf.

**3.** Stir in spinach; cook 5 minutes, stirring frequently. Season with additional salt and black pepper.

**MAKES 4 SERVINGS**

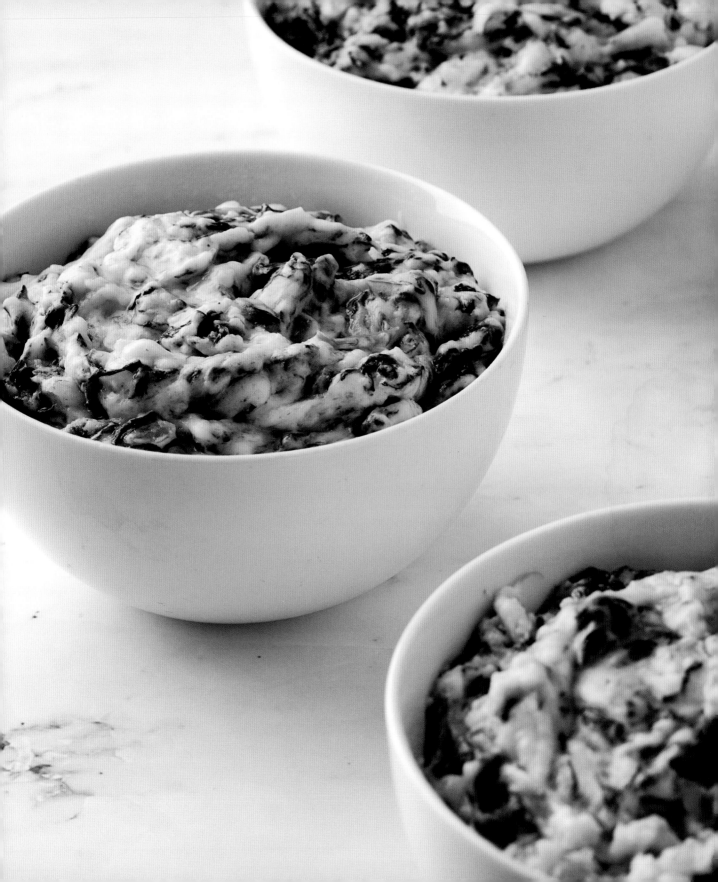

# CRISPY SMASHED POTATOES

- **1 tablespoon plus ½ teaspoon salt, divided**
- **3 pounds unpeeled small red potatoes (2 inches or smaller)**
- **4 tablespoons (½ stick) butter, melted, divided**
- **¼ teaspoon black pepper**
- **½ cup grated Parmesan cheese (optional)**

**1.** Fill large saucepan with water; add 1 tablespoon salt. Bring to a boil over high heat. Add potatoes; boil about 20 minutes or until potatoes are tender when pierced with tip of sharp knife. Drain potatoes; set aside until cool enough to handle.

**2.** Preheat oven to 450°F. Brush baking sheet with 2 tablespoons butter. Working with one potato at a time, smash with hand or bottom of measuring cup to about ½-inch thickness. Arrange smashed potatoes in single layer on prepared baking sheet. Brush with remaining 2 tablespoons butter; sprinkle with remaining ½ teaspoon salt and pepper.

**3.** Bake 30 to 40 minutes or until bottoms of potatoes are golden brown. Turn potatoes; bake 10 minutes. Sprinkle with cheese, if desired; bake 5 minutes or until cheese is melted.

**MAKES ABOUT 6 SERVINGS**

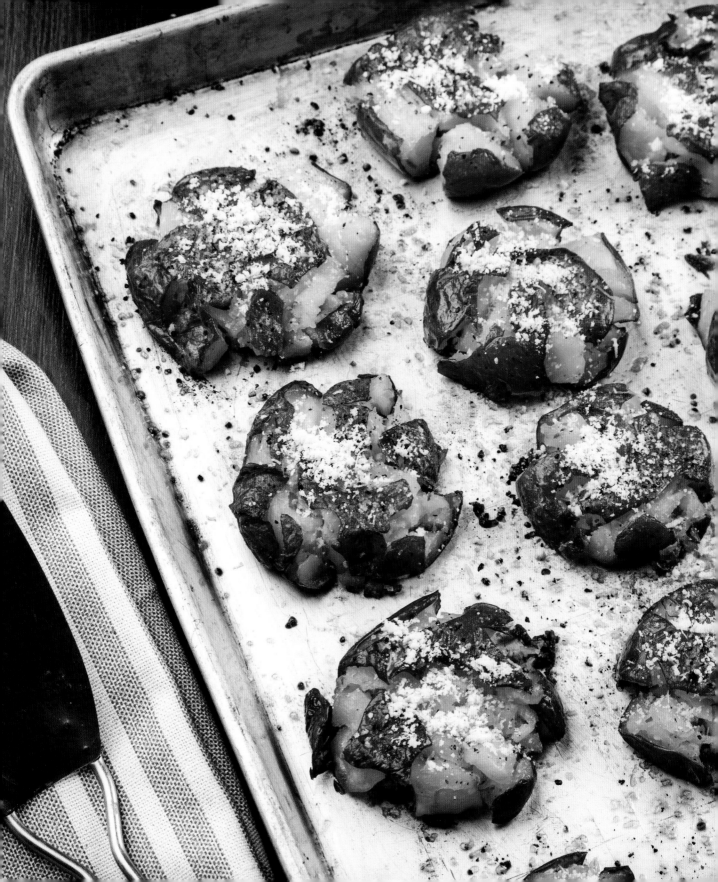

# EXOTIC VEGGIE CHIPS

3 tropical tubers
(malanga, yautia, lila
and/or taro roots)*

1 to 2 green (unripe)
plantains

2 parsnips, peeled

1 medium sweet potato,
peeled

1 lotus root**

Vegetable oil, for deep
frying

Salt

*These tropical tubers
are all similar and their
labels are frequently
interchangeable or
overlapping. They are
available in the produce
section of Latin markets.
Choose whichever tubers
are available and fresh.
Look for firm roots without
signs of mildew or soft
spots.

**Lotus root is available
in the produce section
of Asian markets. The
outside looks like a fat
beige link sausage, but
when sliced, the lacy,
snowflake-like pattern
inside is revealed.

1. Line baking sheets with paper towels.

2. Peel thick shaggy skin from tubers, rinse and
dry. Thinly slice tubers and place in single layer on
prepared baking sheets to absorb excess moisture.
(Stack in multiple layers with paper towels between
layers.) Peel thick skin from plantain. Slice and
place on paper towels. Slice parsnips and sweet
potato and place on paper towels. Trim lotus root
and remove tough skin with paring knife. Slice and
place on paper towels.

3. Fill deep fryer or large heavy skillet with 3 inches
of oil; heat to 350°F on deep-fry thermometer.
Working in batches, fry each vegetable until crisp
and slightly curled, stirring occasionally. (Frying
time will vary from 2 to 6 minutes depending on the
vegetable.)

4. Remove vegetables with slotted spoon and
drain on paper towels; immediately sprinkle with
salt. Cool completely. Store in airtight containers at
room temperature.

**MAKES ABOUT 6 SERVINGS**

TIP

To recrisp chips, bake in preheated 350°F oven
5 minutes.

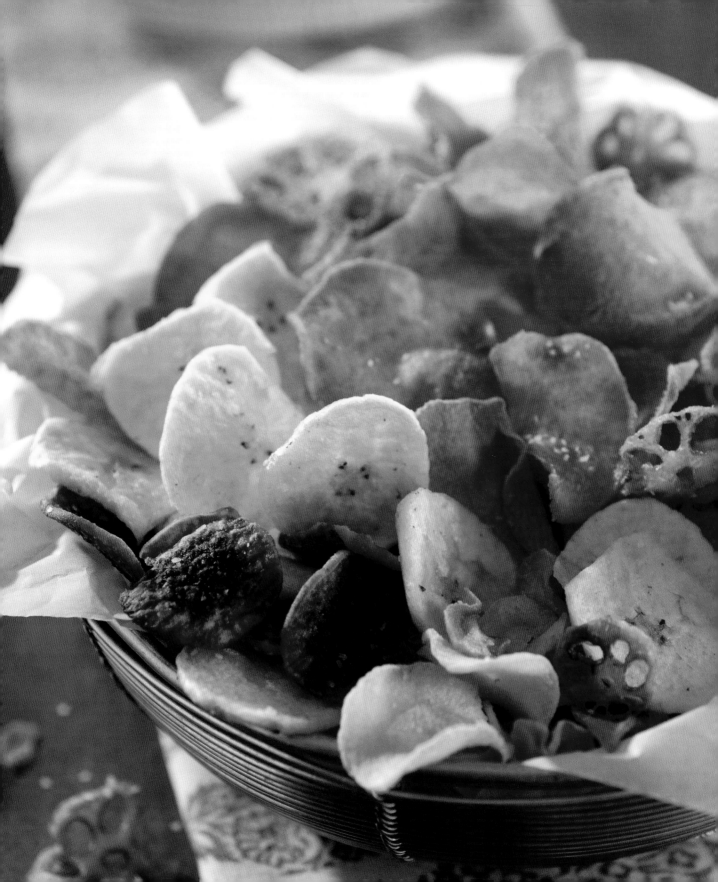

# POTATO CAKES WITH BRUSSELS SPROUTS

2½  **pounds Yukon Gold potatoes, peeled and cut into 1-inch cubes**

6  **tablespoons (¾ stick) butter, melted**

⅓  **cup milk, warmed**

2  **teaspoons salt**

½  **teaspoon black pepper**

3  **tablespoons vegetable oil, divided**

12  **ounces brussels sprouts, ends trimmed, thinly sliced**

4  **green onions, thinly sliced on the diagonal**

1. Place potatoes in large saucepan or Dutch oven; add cold water to cover by 2 inches. Bring to a boil over high heat. Reduce heat to medium-low; cover and simmer about 10 minutes or until potatoes are tender. Drain.

2. Return potatoes to saucepan; mash with potato masher until slightly chunky. Stir in butter, milk, salt and pepper until well blended; set aside.

3. Heat 1 tablespoon oil in large nonstick skillet over medium-high heat. Add brussels sprouts; cook about 8 minutes or until tender and lightly browned, stirring occasionally. Stir brussels sprouts and green onions into potato mixture. Wipe out skillet with paper towel.

4. Heat 1 tablespoon oil in skillet over medium heat. Drop potato mixture into skillet by ½ cupfuls, spacing about ½ inch apart. Cook about 3 minutes per side or until cakes are browned and crisp, pressing down lightly with spatula. Transfer to platter; tent with foil to keep warm. Repeat with remaining 1 tablespoon oil and potato mixture.

**MAKES 12 CAKES**

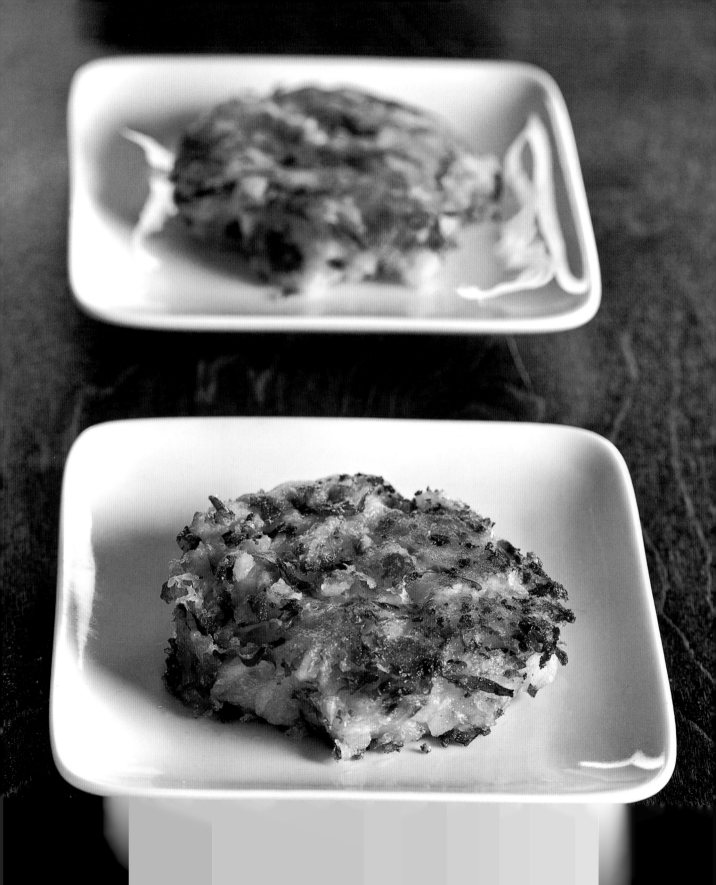

# BAKED TOMATOES WITH CORN BREAD TOPPING

½ cup dry corn bread stuffing mix

¼ cup plus 1 tablespoon grated Parmesan cheese, divided

2 tablespoons minced fresh chives

2 tablespoons minced fresh parsley

¼ teaspoon salt

¼ teaspoon black pepper

1 tablespoon butter

1 shallot, minced

1 clove garlic, minced

4 small to medium tomatoes, halved lengthwise

1. Preheat oven to 350°F. Combine stuffing mix, ¼ cup cheese, chives, parsley, salt and pepper in medium bowl.

2. Melt butter in small skillet over medium heat. Add shallot and garlic; cook and stir 2 minutes or until tender. Stir in stuffing mixture; remove from heat.

3. Arrange tomato halves, cut sides up, in 9-inch round glass pie dish. Spoon topping mixture evenly into each tomato half; sprinkle with remaining 1 tablespoon cheese. Bake 20 minutes or until tomatoes are tender and topping is golden.

**MAKES 8 SERVINGS**

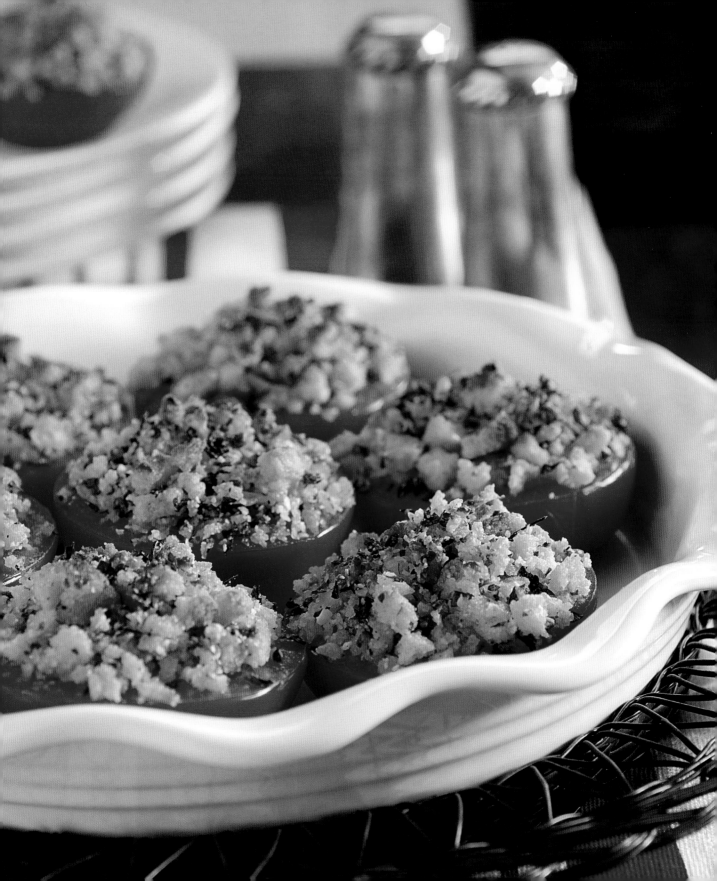

# BROCCOLI AND CHEESE

2 **medium crowns broccoli (1½ pounds), cut into florets (about 6½ cups)**

2 **tablespoons butter**

2 **tablespoons all-purpose flour**

1½ **cups milk**

½ **teaspoon salt**

⅛ **teaspoon ground nutmeg**

⅛ **teaspoon ground red pepper**

1 **cup (4 ounces) shredded Cheddar cheese**

½ **cup (2 ounces) shredded Monterey Jack cheese**

¼ **cup shredded Parmesan cheese**

**Paprika (optional)**

**1.** Bring large saucepan of water to a boil over medium-high heat. Add broccoli; cook 4 to 6 minutes or until tender.

**2.** Meanwhile, melt butter in medium saucepan over medium-high heat. Add flour; whisk until smooth. Gradually whisk in milk until well blended. Cook 2 minutes or until thickened, whisking frequently. Stir in salt, nutmeg and red pepper. Reduce heat to low; whisk in cheeses in three additions, whisking well after first two additions and stirring just until blended after last addition.

**3.** Drain broccoli; place on serving plates. Top with cheese sauce; garnish with paprika. Serve immediately.

**MAKES 4 TO 6 SERVINGS**

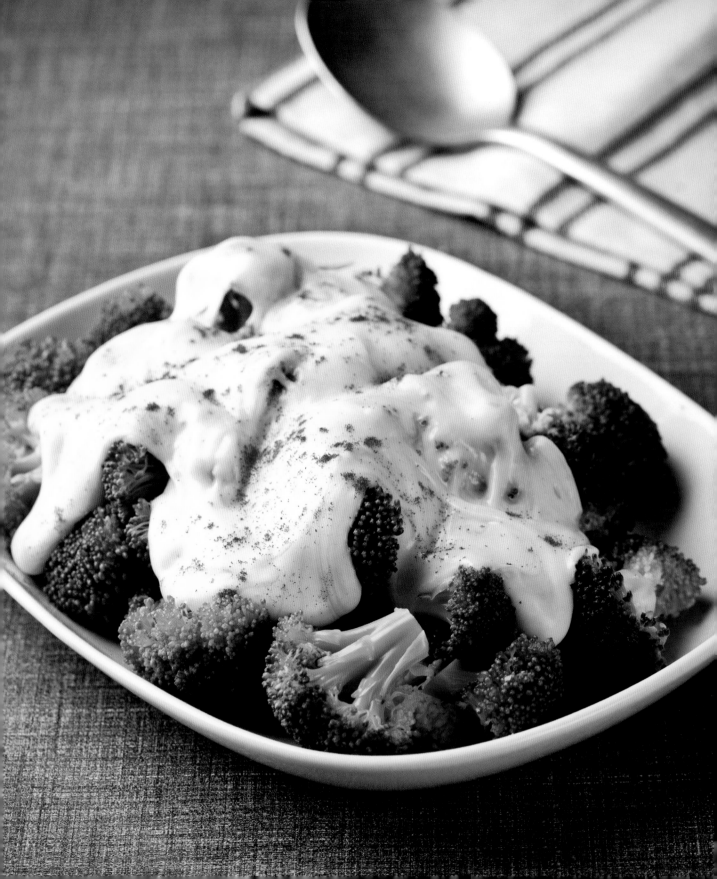

# BALSAMIC BUTTERNUT SQUASH

**3** tablespoons olive oil

**2** tablespoons thinly sliced fresh sage (about 6 large leaves), divided

**1** medium butternut squash, peeled and cut into 1-inch pieces (4 to 5 cups)

**½** red onion, halved and cut into ¼-inch slices

**1** teaspoon salt, divided

**2½** tablespoons balsamic vinegar

**¼** teaspoon black pepper

**1.** Heat oil in large (12-inch) cast iron skillet over medium-high heat. Add 1 tablespoon sage; cook and stir 3 minutes. Add squash, onion and ½ teaspoon salt; cook 6 minutes, stirring occasionally. Reduce heat to medium; cook 15 minutes without stirring.

**2.** Stir in vinegar, remaining ½ teaspoon salt and pepper; cook 10 minutes or until squash is tender, stirring occasionally. Stir in remaining 1 tablespoon sage; cook 1 minute.

**MAKES 4 SERVINGS**

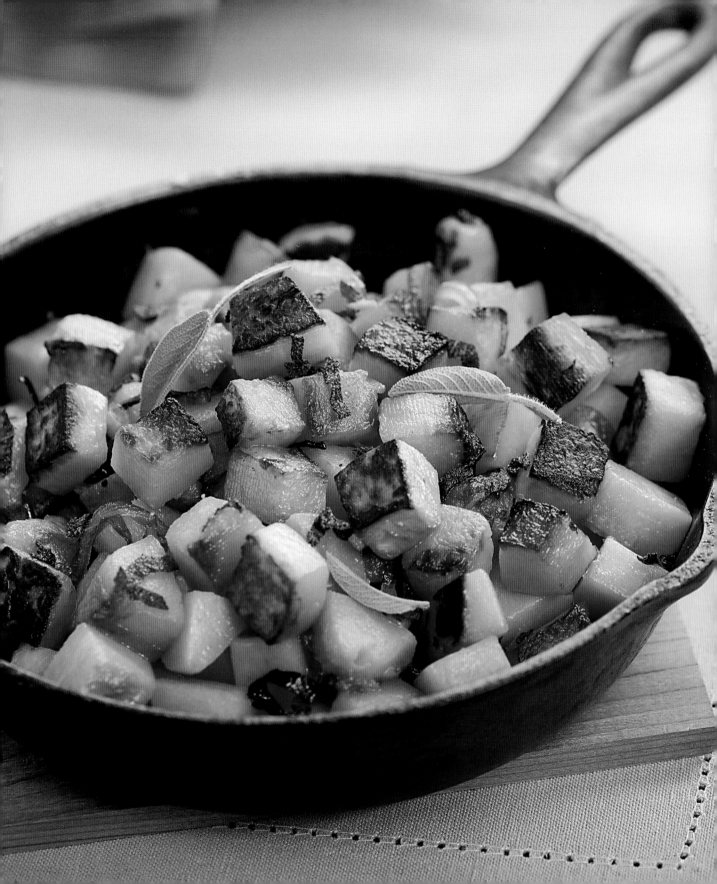

# BOXTY PANCAKES

2 medium russet
   potatoes (1 pound),
   peeled, divided
⅔ cup all-purpose flour
1 teaspoon baking
   powder
½ teaspoon salt
⅔ cup buttermilk
3 tablespoons butter

**1.** Cut 1 potato into 1-inch chunks; place in small saucepan and add cold water to cover by 2 inches. Bring to a boil over medium-high heat; cook 14 to 18 minutes or until tender. Drain potato; return to saucepan and mash. Transfer to medium bowl.

**2.** Grate remaining potato on large holes of box grater; add to bowl with mashed potato. Stir in flour, baking powder and salt until blended. Stir in buttermilk.

**3.** Melt 1 tablespoon butter in large nonstick skillet over medium heat. Drop four slightly heaping tablespoonfuls of batter into skillet; flatten into 2½-inch circles. Cook about 4 minutes per side or until golden and puffed. Remove to plate; cover to keep warm. Repeat with remaining batter and butter. Serve immediately.

**MAKES 4 SERVINGS (16 TO 20 PANCAKES)**

TIP

Serve with melted butter, sour cream or maple syrup.

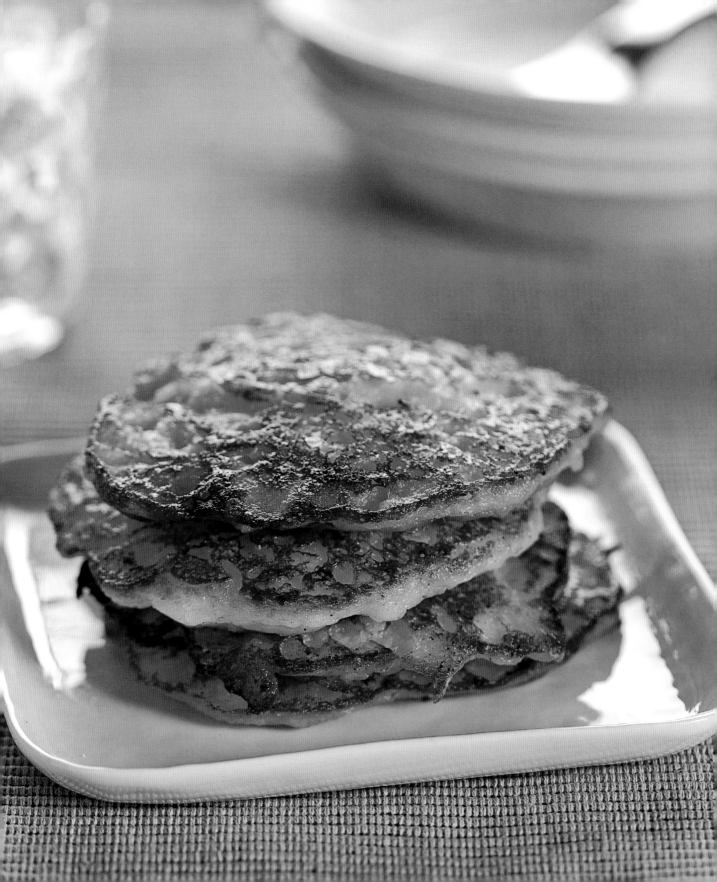

# SWEET POTATO AND APPLE CASSEROLE

- **1 cup all-purpose flour**
- **¾ cup (1½ sticks) butter, melted, divided**
- **½ cup packed brown sugar**
- **½ teaspoon salt**
- **½ teaspoon ground cinnamon**
- **¼ teaspoon ground nutmeg or mace**
- **¼ teaspoon ground cardamom**
- **2 pounds sweet potatoes, peeled, halved lengthwise and thinly sliced**
- **2 Granny Smith apples, peeled, cored, halved lengthwise and thinly sliced**

**1.** Preheat oven to 375°F. Spray 2-quart baking dish with nonstick cooking spray.

**2.** Combine flour, ½ cup butter, brown sugar, ½ teaspoon salt, cinnamon, nutmeg and cardamom in medium bowl until well blended.

**3.** Arrange sweet potatoes and apples in prepared baking dish. Drizzle with remaining ¼ cup butter; season lightly with additional salt.

**4.** Crumble topping over sweet potatoes and apples. Bake 35 to 40 minutes or until topping is brown and potatoes and apples are tender.

**MAKES 8 SERVINGS**

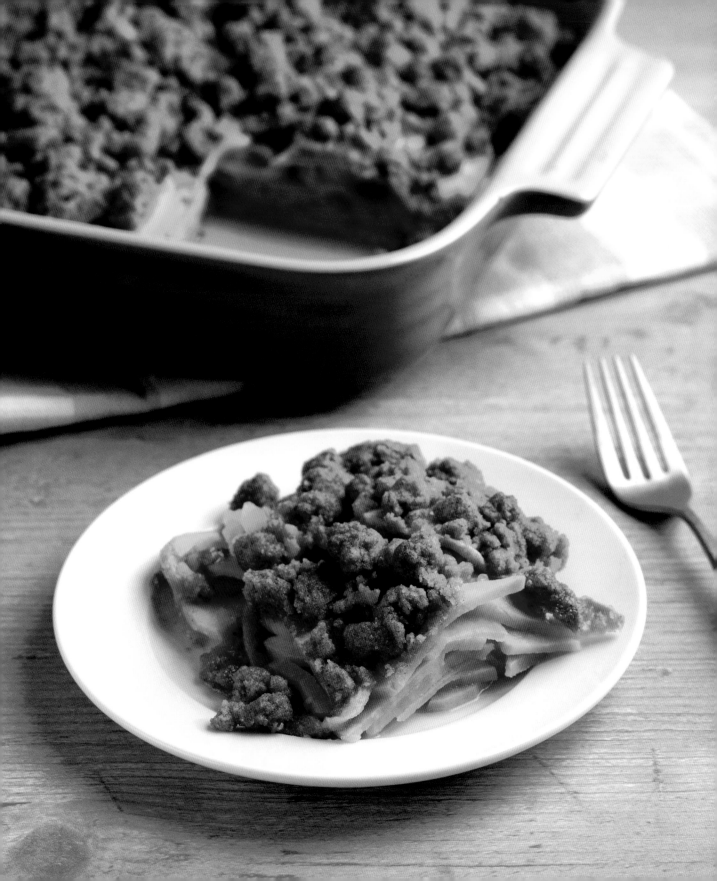

# GREEN BEAN POTATO SALAD

½ **cup thinly sliced red onion**

¼ **cup plus 2 tablespoons white wine vinegar, divided**

2 **tablespoons water**

1 **teaspoon sugar**

1½ **teaspoons salt, divided**

2 **cups cubed assorted potatoes (purple, baby red, Yukon Gold and/or a combination)**

1 **cup cut fresh green beans (1-inch pieces)**

2 **tablespoons plain Greek yogurt**

2 **tablespoons olive oil**

1 **tablespoon spicy mustard**

1. Combine red onion, ¼ cup vinegar, 2 tablespoons water, sugar and ½ teaspoon salt in large glass jar. Seal jar; shake well. Refrigerate at least 1 hour or up to 1 week.

2. Bring large saucepan of water to a boil. Add potatoes; cook 5 to 8 minutes or until fork-tender. Add green beans during last 4 minutes of cooking time. Drain potatoes and green beans.

3. Whisk yogurt, remaining 2 tablespoons vinegar, oil, mustard and remaining ½ teaspoon salt in large bowl until smooth and well blended.

4. Add potatoes and green beans to dressing. Drain onions; add to bowl with potatoes. Toss gently to coat. Cover and refrigerate at least 1 hour before serving to allow flavors to develop.

**MAKES 6 SERVINGS**

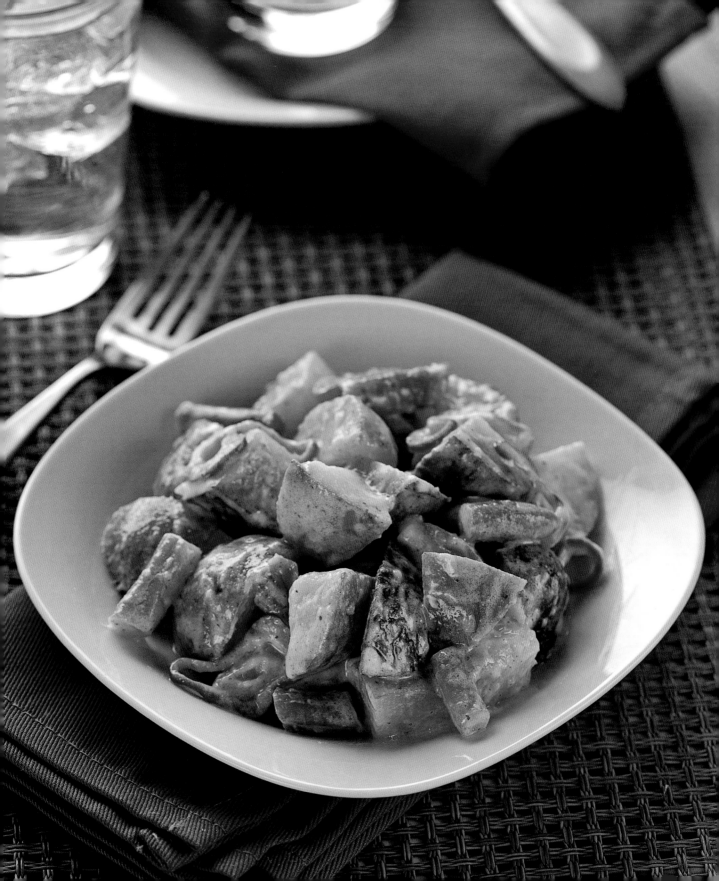

# CREAMY COLESLAW

½ **cup mayonnaise**

½ **cup buttermilk**

2 **teaspoons sugar**

1 **teaspoon celery seed**

1 **teaspoon fresh lime juice**

½ **teaspoon chili powder**

3 **cups shredded coleslaw mix**

1 **cup shredded carrots**

¼ **cup finely chopped red onion**

**1.** Whisk mayonnaise, buttermilk, sugar, celery seed, lime juice and chili powder in large bowl until smooth and well blended. Add coleslaw mix, carrots and onion; toss to coat evenly.

**2.** Cover and refrigerate at least 2 hours before serving.

**MAKES 4 SERVINGS**

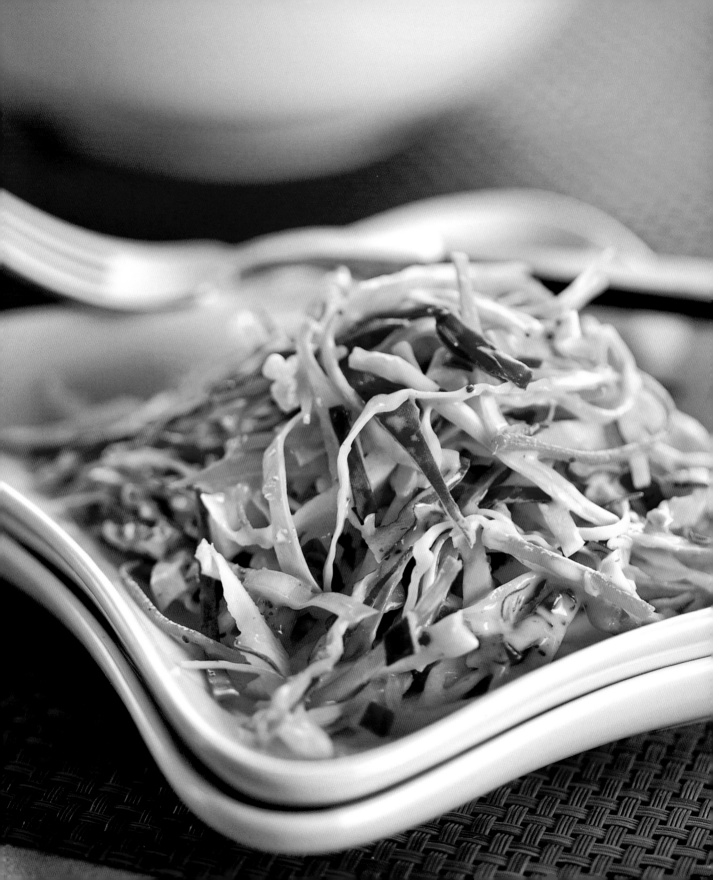

# CORN FRITTERS

2 large ears corn

2 eggs, separated

¼ cup all-purpose flour

1 tablespoon sugar

1 tablespoon butter, melted

¼ teaspoon salt

⅛ teaspoon black pepper

⅛ teaspoon cream of tartar

1 to 2 tablespoons vegetable oil

1. Husk corn. Cut kernels from ears (1½ to 2 cups); place in medium bowl. Hold cobs over bowl, scraping with back of knife to extract juice. Transfer about half of kernels to food processor; process 2 to 3 seconds or until coarsely chopped. Add to whole kernels.

2. Whisk egg yolks in large bowl. Whisk in flour, sugar, butter, salt and pepper. Stir in corn mixture.

3. Beat egg whites and cream of tartar in separate large bowl with electric mixer at high speed until stiff peaks form. Fold egg whites into corn mixture.

4. Heat 1 tablespoon oil in 12-inch nonstick skillet over medium-high heat. Drop ¼ cupfuls of batter into skillet 1-inch apart. Cook 3 to 5 minutes per side or until lightly browned. Repeat with remaining batter, adding more oil, if necessary. Serve hot.

**MAKES 8 TO 9 FRITTERS**

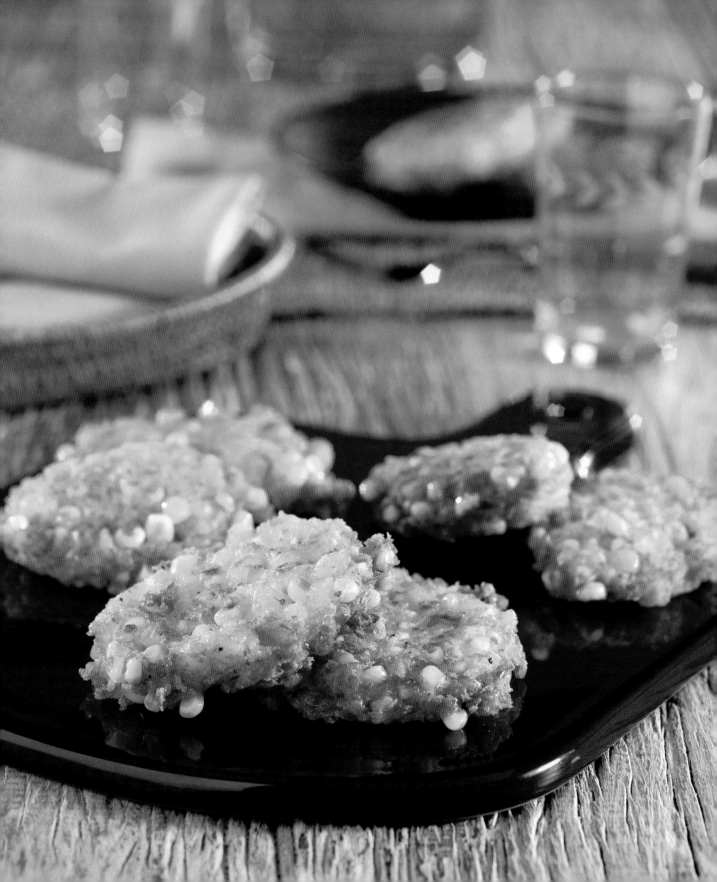

# BRAISED BRUSSELS SPROUTS WITH CARAMELIZED ONIONS

1 **pound brussels sprouts, trimmed and halved lengthwise**

1 **tablespoon butter**

1 **cup chopped onion**

2 **tablespoons honey or molasses, divided**

1 **tablespoon balsamic vinegar**

3 **tablespoons dry white wine, divided**

**Salt and black pepper**

**1.** Bring medium saucepan of water to a boil. Add brussels sprouts; cook 5 minutes. Drain.

**2.** Heat butter in large skillet over medium-low heat. Add onion; cook and stir 10 minutes or until tender and lightly browned. Add 1 tablespoon honey and vinegar; cook 5 minutes.

**3.** Add brussels sprouts to skillet with onions and increase heat to medium. Add 2 tablespoons wine and remaining 1 tablespoon honey; cook about 3 minutes or until most liquid has evaporated.

**4.** Add remaining 1 tablespoon wine to skillet; cook and stir  2 minutes or until brussels sprouts are tender. Season with salt and pepper.

**MAKES 4 SERVINGS**

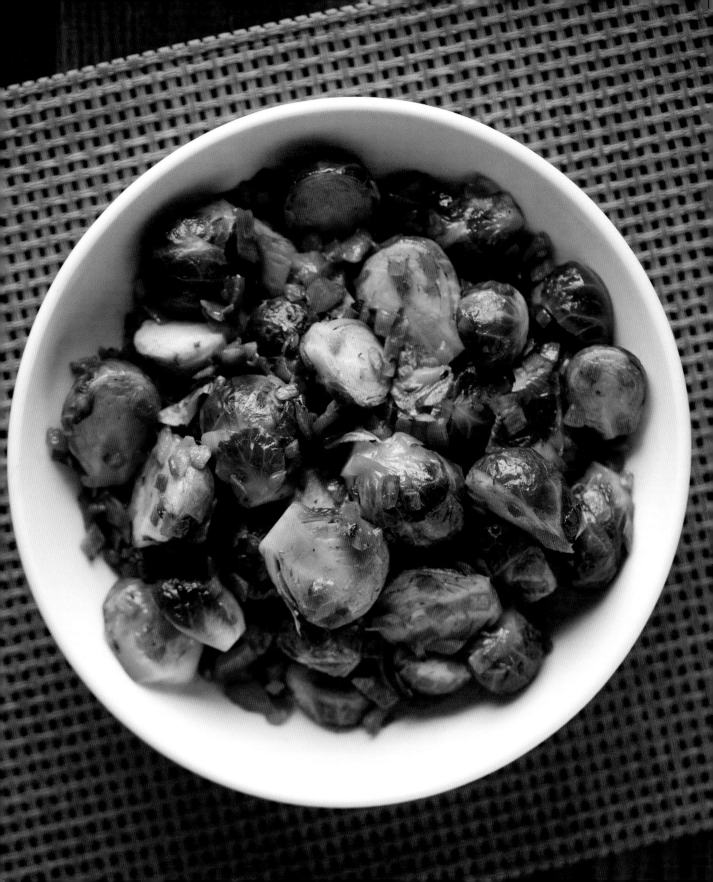

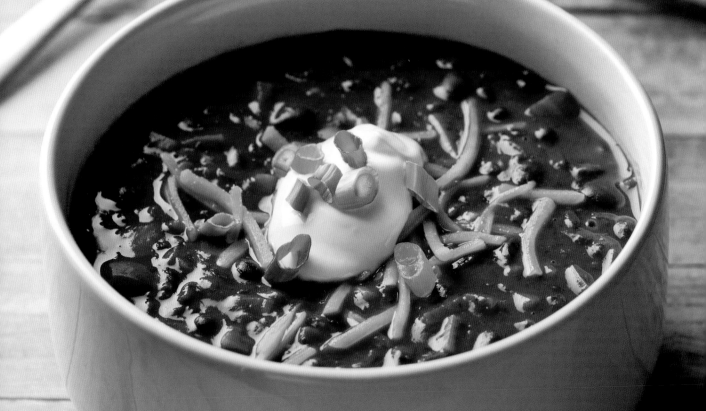

# CHAPTER 6
# SOUPS & CHILIS

# BLACK BEAN SOUP

- 2 tablespoons vegetable oil
- 1 cup diced onion
- 1 stalk celery, diced
- 2 carrots, diced
- ½ small green bell pepper, diced
- 4 cloves garlic, minced
- 4 cans (15 ounces each) black beans, rinsed and drained, divided
- 4 cups (32 ounces) vegetable broth, divided
- 2 tablespoons cider vinegar
- 2 teaspoons chili powder
- ½ teaspoon salt
- ½ teaspoon ground red pepper
- ½ teaspoon ground cumin
- ¼ teaspoon liquid smoke
- Garnishes: sour cream, chopped green onions and shredded Cheddar cheese

**1.** Heat oil in large saucepan or Dutch oven over medium-low heat. Add onion, celery, carrots, bell pepper and garlic; cook 10 minutes, stirring occasionally.

**2.** Combine half of beans and 1 cup broth in food processor or blender; process until smooth. Add to vegetables in saucepan.

**3.** Stir in remaining beans, remaining broth, vinegar, chili powder, salt, red pepper, cumin and liquid smoke; bring to a boil over high heat. Reduce heat to medium-low; simmer 1 hour or until vegetables are tender and soup is thickened. Garnish as desired.

**MAKES 4 TO 6 SERVINGS**

# GARDEN VEGETABLE SOUP

- 1 tablespoon olive oil
- 1 medium onion, chopped
- 1 carrot, chopped
- 1 stalk celery, chopped
- 1 medium zucchini, diced
- 1 medium yellow squash, diced
- 1 red bell pepper, diced
- 2 tablespoons tomato paste
- 2 cloves garlic, minced
- 2 teaspoons salt
- 1 teaspoon Italian seasoning
- ½ teaspoon black pepper
- 8 cups vegetable broth
- 1 can (28 ounces) whole tomatoes, chopped, juice reserved
- ½ cup uncooked pearl barley
- 1 cup cut green beans (1-inch pieces)
- ½ cup corn
- ¼ cup slivered fresh basil
- 1 tablespoon lemon juice

**1.** Heat oil in large saucepan or Dutch oven over medium-high heat. Add onion, carrot and celery; cook and stir 8 minutes or until vegetables are softened. Add zucchini, yellow squash and bell pepper; cook and stir 5 minutes or until softened. Stir in tomato paste, garlic, salt, Italian seasoning and black pepper; cook 1 minute. Stir in broth and tomatoes with juice; bring to a boil. Stir in barley.

**2.** Reduce heat to low; simmer 30 minutes. Stir in green beans and corn; cook about 15 minutes or until barley is tender and green beans are crisp-tender. Stir in basil and lemon juice.

**MAKES 8 TO 10 SERVINGS**

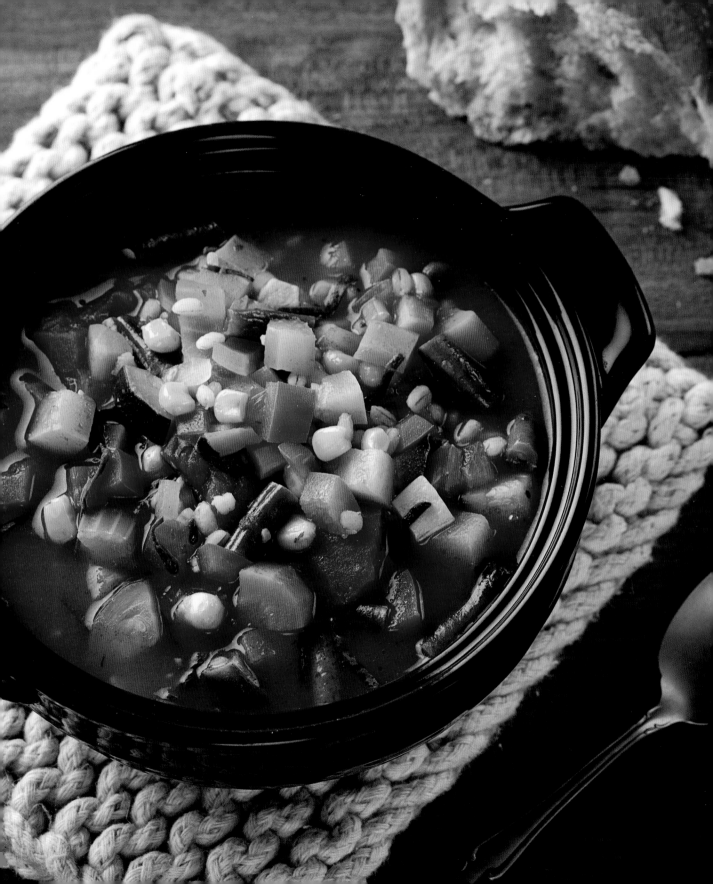

# CREAMY TOMATO SOUP

- **3** **tablespoons olive oil, divided**
- **2** **tablespoons butter**
- **1** **large onion, finely chopped**
- **2** **cloves garlic, minced**
- **2** **teaspoons sugar**
- **1** **teaspoon salt**
- **½** **teaspoon dried oregano**
- **2** **cans (28 ounces each) peeled Italian plum tomatoes, undrained**
- **4** **cups ½-inch focaccia cubes (half of 9-ounce loaf)**
- **½** **teaspoon black pepper**
- **½** **cup whipping cream**

**1.** Heat 2 tablespoons oil and butter in large saucepan over medium-high heat. Add onion; cook and stir 5 minutes or until softened. Add garlic, sugar, salt and oregano; cook 30 seconds. Stir in tomatoes with juice; bring to a boil. Reduce heat to medium-low; simmer 45 minutes, stirring occasionally.

**2.** Meanwhile, prepare croutons. Preheat oven to 350°F. Combine focaccia cubes, remaining 1 tablespoon oil and pepper in large bowl; toss to coat. Spread on large rimmed baking sheet. Bake about 10 minutes or until bread cubes are golden brown.

**3.** Blend soup with immersion blender until smooth. (Or process in batches in food processor or blender.) Stir in cream; heat through. Serve soup topped with croutons.

**MAKES 6 SERVINGS**

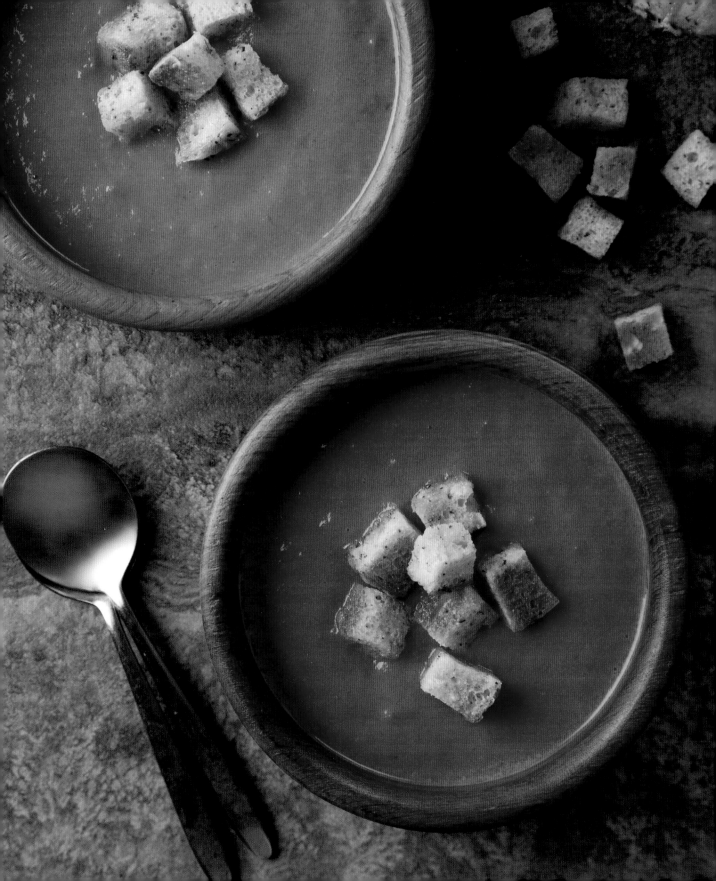

# WEST AFRICAN PEANUT SOUP

2 tablespoons vegetable oil

1 large onion, chopped

½ cup chopped roasted peanuts

1½ tablespoons minced fresh ginger

4 cloves garlic, minced

1 teaspoon salt

4 cups vegetable broth

2 sweet potatoes, peeled and cut into ½-inch cubes

1 can (28 ounces) whole tomatoes, drained and coarsely chopped

¼ teaspoon ground red pepper

1 bunch Swiss chard or kale, stemmed and thinly sliced

⅓ cup unsweetened peanut butter (creamy or chunky)

**1.** Heat oil in large saucepan over medium-high heat. Add onion; cook and stir 5 minutes or until softened. Add peanuts, ginger, garlic and salt; cook and stir 1 minute. Stir in broth, sweet potatoes, tomatoes and red pepper; bring to a boil. Reduce heat to medium; simmer 10 minutes.

**2.** Stir in kale and peanut butter; cook over medium-low heat 10 minutes or until vegetables are tender and soup is creamy.

**MAKES 6 TO 8 SERVINGS**

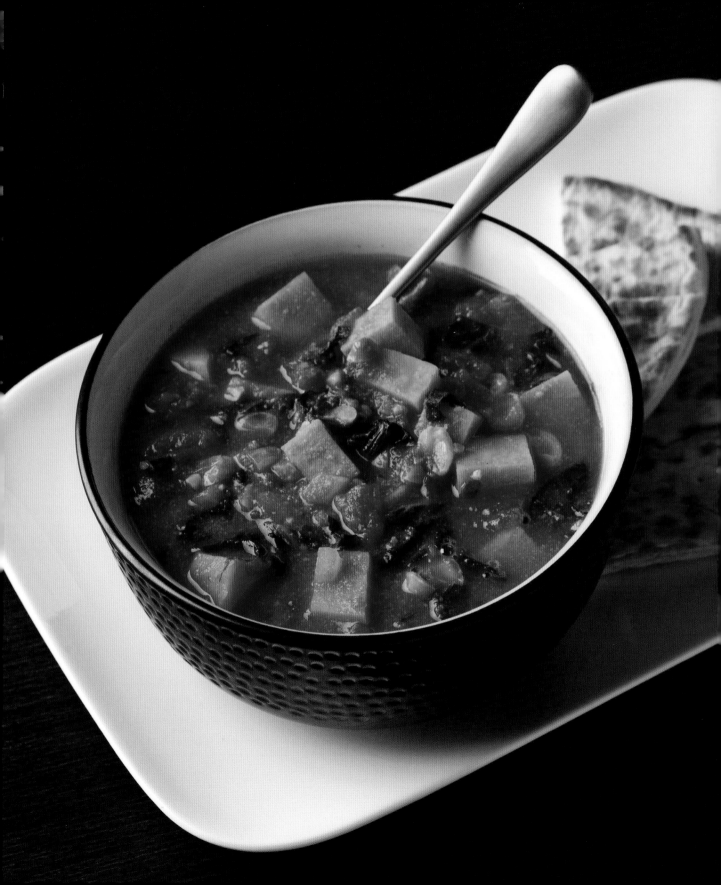

# RAINBOW VEGETABLE STEW

- 1 tablespoon olive oil
- 1 red onion, chopped
- 2 stalks celery, chopped
- 3 cloves garlic, minced
- 2 teaspoons salt, divided
- 4 cups vegetable broth
- 1 butternut squash (about 2 pounds), peeled and cut into ½-inch cubes
- 1 red bell pepper, chopped
- 1 green bell pepper, chopped
- 1 teaspoon ground cumin
- ½ teaspoon dried oregano
- ¼ teaspoon ground chipotle pepper
- 1½ cups water
- ¾ cup uncooked tricolor or white quinoa, rinsed well in fine-mesh strainer
- ½ cup corn
- 1 can (15 ounces) black beans, rinsed and drained
- ½ cup chopped fresh parsley
- 1 tablespoon lime juice

**1.** Heat oil in large saucepan over medium-high heat. Add onion and celery; cook and stir 5 minutes or until vegetables are softened. Add garlic and 1½ teaspoons salt; cook and stir 30 seconds. Stir in broth, squash, bell peppers, cumin, oregano and chipotle pepper; bring to a boil. Reduce heat to medium; simmer 20 minutes or until squash is tender.

**2.** Meanwhile, bring 1½ cups water, quinoa and remaining ½ teaspoon salt to a boil in medium saucepan. Reduce heat to low; cover and simmer 15 minutes or until quinoa is tender and water is absorbed.

**3.** Stir corn and beans into stew; cook 5 minutes or until heated through. Stir in parsley and lime juice. Serve with quinoa.

**MAKES 4 TO 6 SERVINGS**

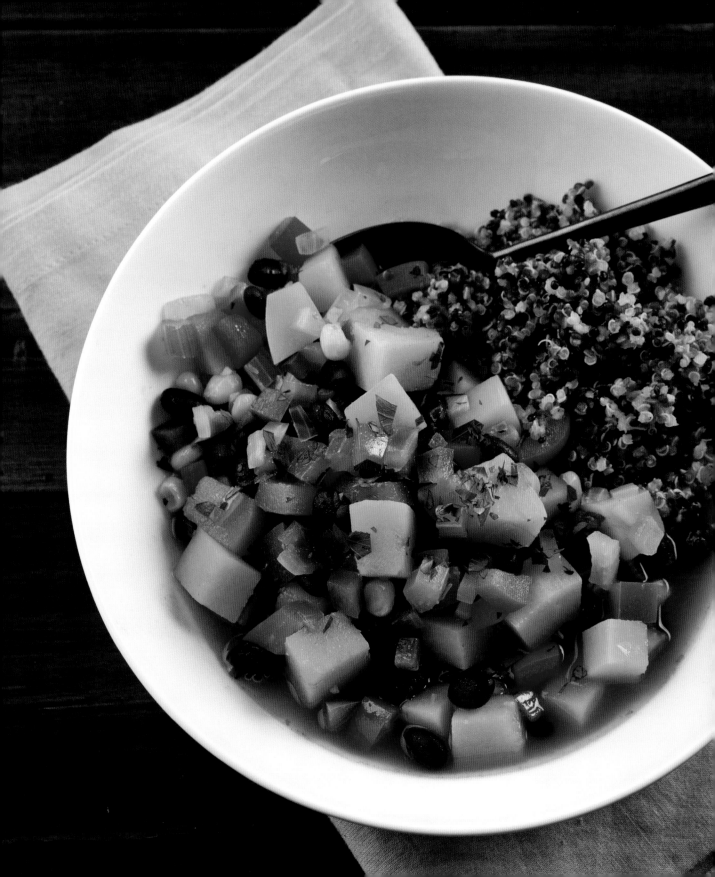

# CLASSIC LENTIL SOUP

- **2** tablespoons olive oil, divided
- **2** medium onions, chopped
- **1½** teaspoons salt
- **4** cloves garlic, minced
- **¼** cup tomato paste
- **1** teaspoon dried oregano
- **½** teaspoon dried basil
- **¼** teaspoon dried thyme
- **¼** teaspoon black pepper
- **½** cup dry sherry or white wine
- **8** cups vegetable broth
- **2** cups water
- **3** carrots, cut into ½-inch pieces
- **2** cups dried lentils, rinsed
- **1** cup chopped fresh parsley
- **1** tablespoon balsamic vinegar

**1.** Heat 1 tablespoon oil in large saucepan or Dutch oven over medium heat. Add onions; cook 10 minutes, stirring occasionally. Add remaining 1 tablespoon oil and salt; cook 10 minutes or until onions are golden brown, stirring frequently.

**2.** Add garlic; cook and stir 1 minute. Add tomato paste, oregano, basil, thyme and pepper; cook and stir 1 minute. Stir in sherry; cook 30 seconds, scraping up browned bits from bottom of saucepan.

**3.** Stir in broth, water, carrots and lentils; cover and bring to a boil over high heat. Reduce heat to medium-low; cook, partially covered, 30 minutes or until lentils are tender.

**4.** Remove from heat; stir in parsley and vinegar.

### MAKES 6 TO 8 SERVINGS

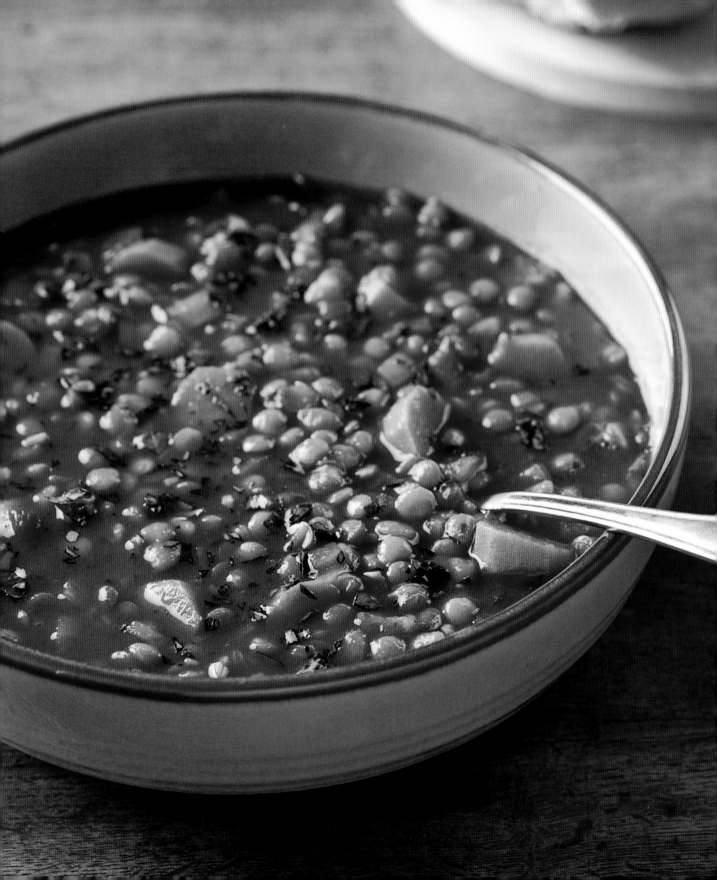

# CORN CHIP CHILI

1 tablespoon olive oil

1 medium onion, chopped

1 medium red bell pepper, chopped

1 jalapeño pepper, seeded and finely chopped

4 cloves garlic, minced

2 pounds refrigerated plant-based ground meatless product *or* 2 packages (10 ounces each) frozen meatless crumbles

1 can (4 ounces) diced green chiles, drained

2 cans (about 14 ounces each) fire-roasted diced tomatoes

2 tablespoons chili powder

1½ teaspoons ground cumin

1½ teaspoons dried oregano

¾ teaspoon salt

3 cups corn chips

Garnishes: shredded sharp Cheddar cheese and sliced green onions

**1.** Heat oil in large saucepan over medium-high heat. Add onion, bell pepper, jalapeño pepper and garlic; cook and stir 3 minutes or until softened. Add meatless product; cook and stir 10 minutes, breaking into crumbles with wooden spoon. Stir in green chiles; cook 1 minute. Stir in tomatoes, chili powder, cumin, oregano and salt. Bring to a boil. Reduce heat to low; simmer, partially covered, 30 minutes.

**2.** Place corn chips in serving bowls; top with chili. Sprinkle with cheese and green onions.

**MAKES 6 SERVINGS**

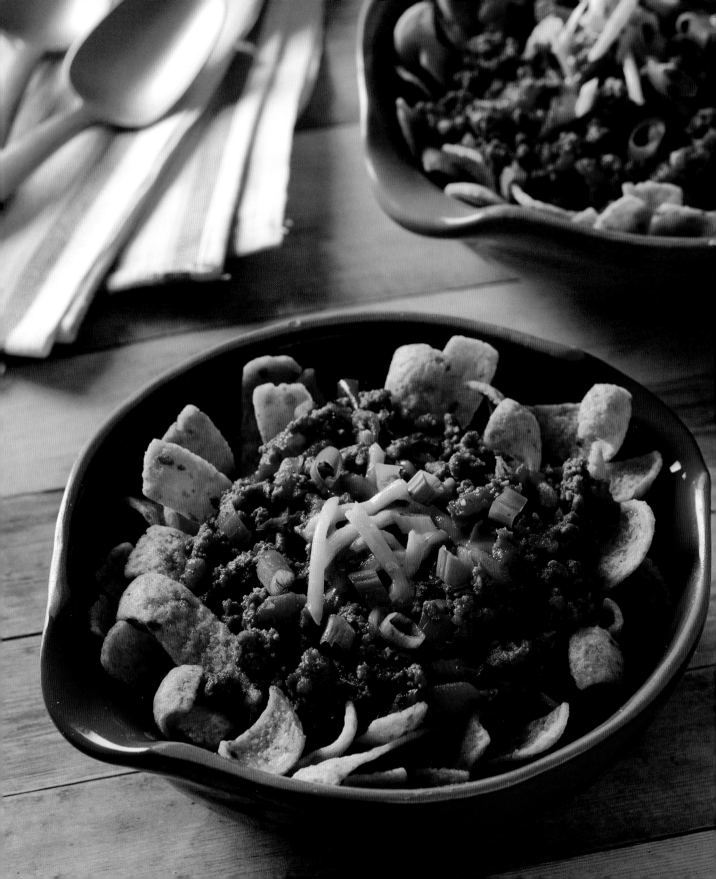

# PASTA E CECI

4 tablespoons olive oil, divided

1 onion, chopped

1 carrot, chopped

1 clove garlic, minced

1 rosemary sprig *or* ½ teaspoon dried rosemary

1 teaspoon salt

1 can (28 ounces) whole tomatoes, drained and crushed

2 cups vegetable broth or water

1 can (15 ounces) chickpeas, undrained

1 bay leaf

⅛ teaspoon red pepper flakes

1 cup uncooked orecchiette or medium shell pasta

Black pepper

Chopped fresh parsley or basil

**1.** Heat 3 tablespoons oil in large saucepan over medium-high heat. Add onion and carrot; cook 10 minutes or until vegetables are softened, stirring occasionally.

**2.** Add garlic, rosemary and salt; cook and stir 1 minute. Stir in tomatoes, broth, chickpeas with liquid, bay leaf and red pepper flakes. Remove 1 cup mixture to food processor or blender; process until smooth. Stir back into saucepan; bring to a boil.

**3.** Stir in pasta. Reduce heat to medium; cook 12 to 15 minutes or until pasta is tender and mixture is creamy. Remove and discard bay leaf and rosemary sprig. Taste and season with additional salt and black pepper, if desired. Divide among bowls; garnish with parsley and drizzle with remaining 1 tablespoon oil.

**MAKES 4 SERVINGS**

TIP

To crush the tomatoes, crush them between your fingers over the pot. Or coarsely chop them with a knife.

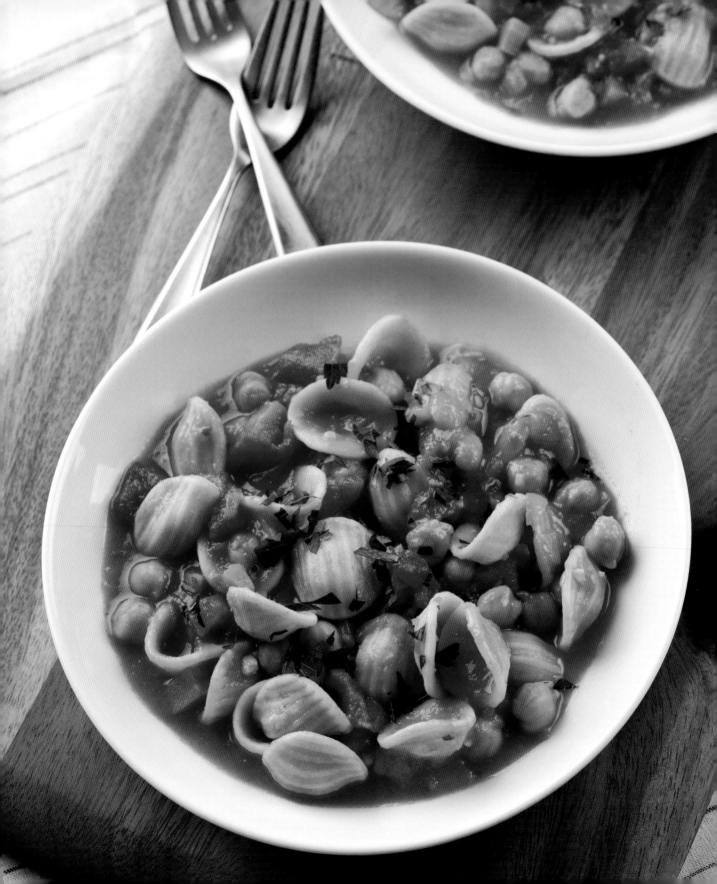

# QUINOA CHILI

2 tablespoons vegetable oil

1 large onion

1 red bell pepper, diced

1 large carrot, peeled and diced

1 stalk celery, diced

1 jalapeño pepper, seeded and finely chopped

1 tablespoon minced garlic

3 tablespoons chili powder

2 teaspoons ground cumin

1 teaspoon salt

1 can (15 ounces) kidney beans, rinsed and drained

1 can (28 ounces) crushed tomatoes

1 cup water

1 cup fresh or frozen corn

½ cup uncooked quinoa, rinsed well in fine-mesh strainer

Garnishes: diced avocado, shredded Cheddar cheese and sliced green onions

**1.** Heat oil in large saucepan over medium-high heat. Add onion, bell pepper, carrot and celery; cook about 10 minutes or until vegetables are softened, stirring occasionally. Add jalapeño pepper, garlic, chili powder, cumin and salt; cook about 1 minute or until fragrant.

**2.** Add beans, tomatoes, water, corn and quinoa; bring to a boil. Reduce heat to low; cover and simmer 1 hour, stirring occasionally.

**3.** Spoon into bowls; garnish as desired.

**MAKES 4 TO 6 SERVINGS**

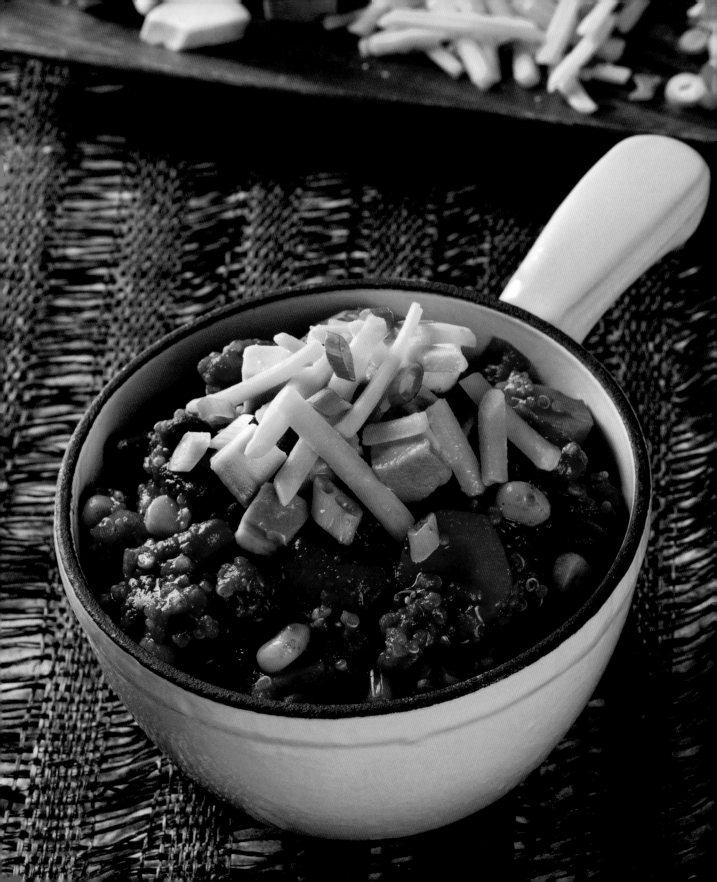

# MINESTRONE SOUP

1 tablespoon olive oil

½ cup chopped onion

1 stalk celery, diced

1 carrot, diced

2 cloves garlic, minced

2 cups vegetable broth

1½ cups water

1 bay leaf

¾ teaspoon salt

½ teaspoon dried basil

½ teaspoon dried oregano

¼ teaspoon dried thyme

¼ teaspoon sugar

Ground black pepper

1 can (15 ounces) dark red kidney beans, rinsed and drained

1 can (15 ounces) navy beans or cannellini beans, rinsed and drained

1 can (about 14 ounces) diced tomatoes

1 cup diced zucchini (about 1 small)

½ cup uncooked small shell pasta

½ cup fresh or frozen cut green beans

¼ cup dry red wine

1 cup packed chopped fresh spinach

**1.** Heat oil in large saucepan or Dutch oven over medium-high heat. Add onion, celery, carrot and garlic; cook and stir 5 to 7 minutes or until vegetables are tender. Add broth, water, bay leaf, salt, basil, oregano, thyme, sugar and pepper; bring to a boil.

**2.** Stir in kidney beans, navy beans, tomatoes, zucchini, pasta, green beans and wine; cook 10 minutes, stirring occasionally.

**3.** Add spinach; cook 2 minutes or until pasta and zucchini are tender. Remove and discard bay leaf before serving.

**MAKES 4 TO 6 SERVINGS**

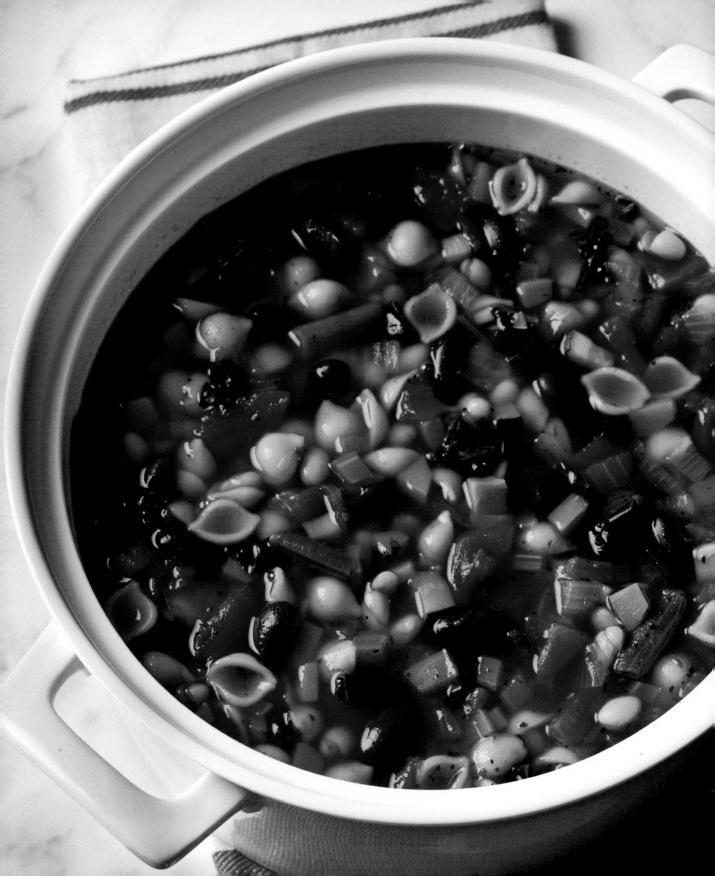

# BROCCOLI CHEESE SOUP

- **6 tablespoons butter**
- **1 cup chopped onion**
- **1 clove garlic, minced**
- **¼ cup all-purpose flour**
- **2 cups vegetable broth**
- **2 cups milk**
- **1½ teaspoons Dijon mustard**
- **½ teaspoon salt**
- **¼ teaspoon ground nutmeg**
- **¼ teaspoon black pepper**
- **⅛ teaspoon hot pepper sauce**
- **1 package (16 ounces) frozen broccoli (5 cups)**
- **2 carrots, shredded (1 cup)**
- **6 ounces pasteurized process cheese product, cubed**
- **1 cup (4 ounces) shredded sharp Cheddar cheese, plus additional for garnish**

**1.** Melt butter in large saucepan or Dutch oven over medium-low heat. Add onion; cook and stir 8 minutes or until softened. Add garlic; cook and stir 1 minute. Increase heat to medium. Whisk in flour until smooth; cook and stir 3 minutes without browning.

**2.** Gradually whisk in broth and milk. Add mustard, salt, nutmeg, black pepper and hot pepper sauce; cook 15 minutes or until thickened, stirring occasionally.

**3.** Add broccoli; cook 15 minutes. Add carrots; cook 10 minutes or until vegetables are tender.

**4.** Transfer half of soup to food processor or blender; process until smooth. Return to saucepan. Add cheese product and 1 cup Cheddar; cook and stir over low heat until cheese is melted. Ladle into bowls; garnish with additional Cheddar.

**MAKES 4 TO 6 SERVINGS**

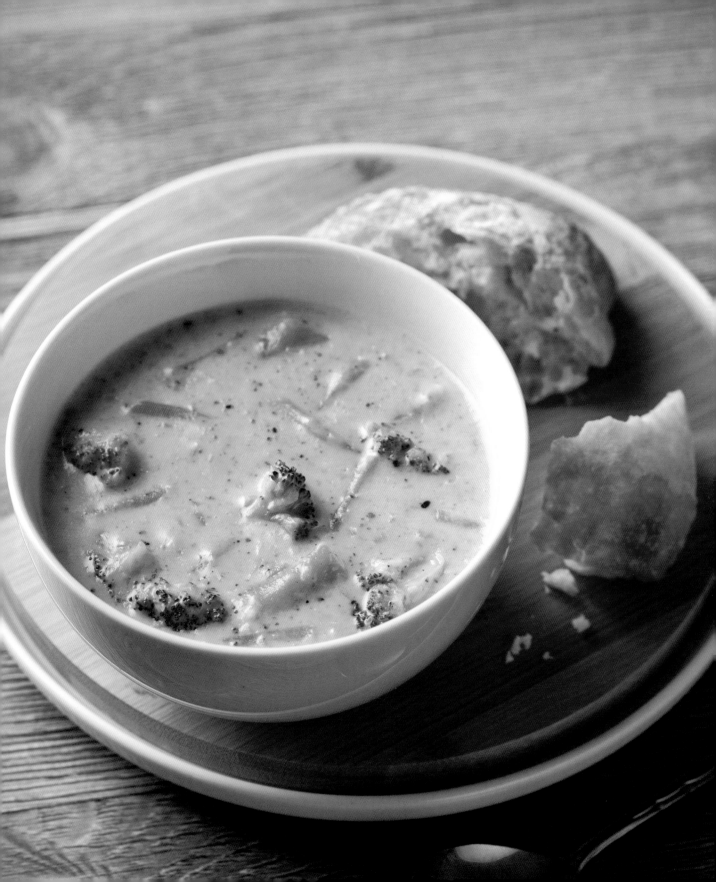

# SWEET POTATO AND BLACK BEAN CHIPOTLE CHILI

1 tablespoon vegetable oil

2 large onions, diced

1 tablespoon minced garlic

2 tablespoons tomato paste

3 tablespoons chili powder

1 tablespoon ground chipotle pepper

1 teaspoon ground cumin

2 teaspoons salt

1 cup water

1 large sweet potato, peeled and cut into ½-inch pieces (about 2 pounds)

2 cans (28 ounces each) black beans, rinsed and drained

2 cans (28 ounces each) crushed tomatoes

Garnishes: sour cream, sliced green onions, shredded cheddar cheese and/or tortilla strips

**1.** Heat oil in large saucepan over medium-high heat. Add onions; cook 8 minutes or until softened and lightly browned. Add garlic, tomato paste, chili powder, chipotle pepper, cumin and salt; cook and stir 1 minute. Add water, stirring to scrape up browned bits from bottom of saucepan.

**2.** Add sweet potatoes, beans and tomatoes; bring to a boil. Reduce heat to low; simmer 30 minutes or until sweet potatoes are tender.

**3.** Ladle into bowls; garnish as desired.

**MAKES 8 TO 10 SERVINGS**

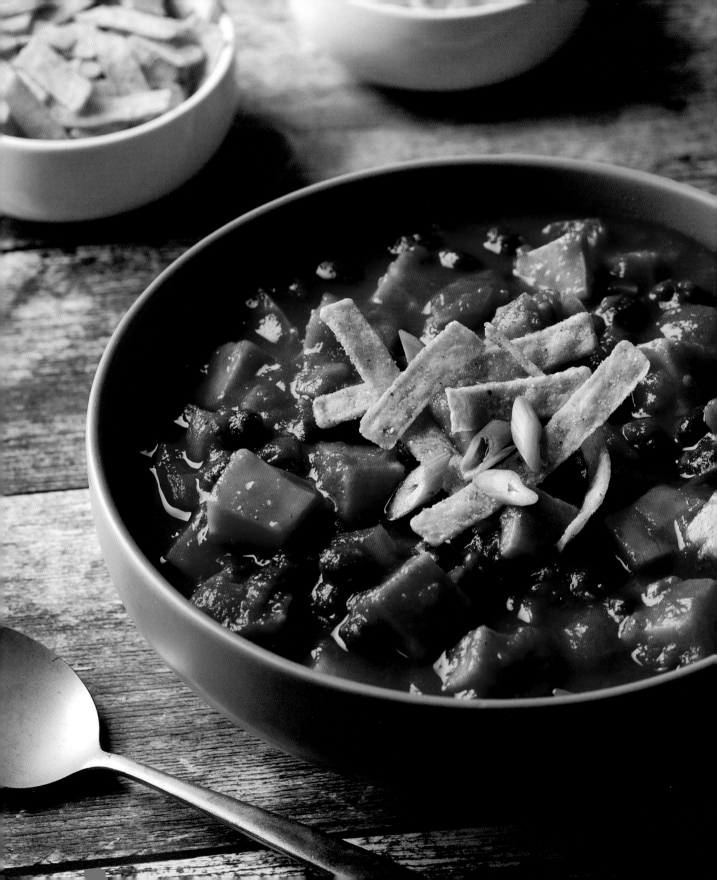

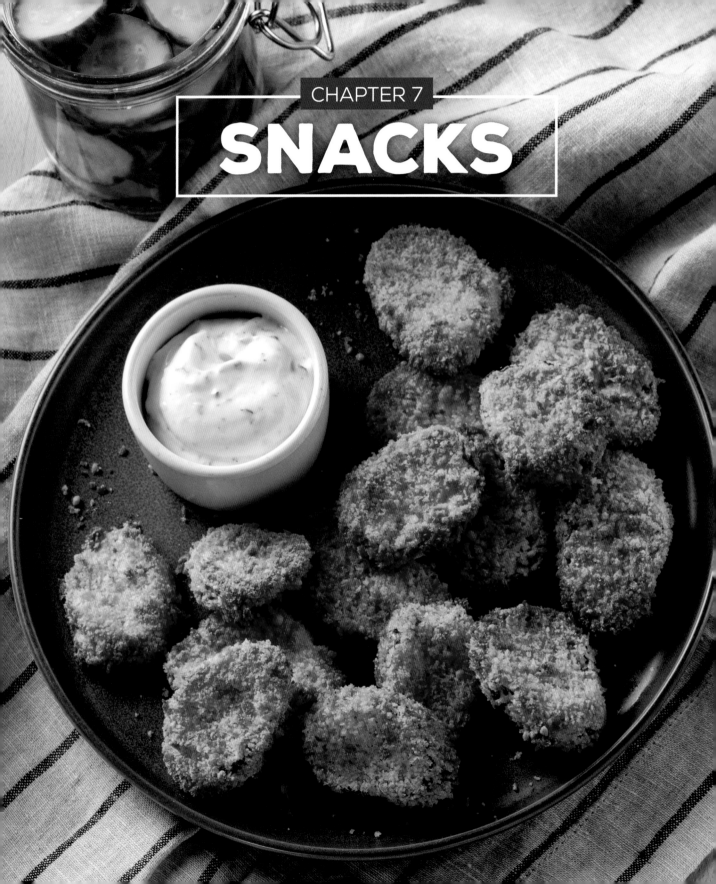

# CHAPTER 7

# SNACKS

# PARMESAN PICKLE CHIPS

4 large whole dill pickles
   (about 5 inches)

½ cup all-purpose flour

½ teaspoon salt

2 eggs

1 cup panko bread
   crumbs

¼ cup grated Parmesan
   cheese

  Garlic aioli,
   mayonnaise or ranch
   dressing for dipping

**1.** Preheat oven to 350°F. Line baking sheet with parchment paper. Line cutting board with paper towels. Slice pickles diagonally into ¼-inch slices, place on paper towels on cutting board. Pat dry with additional paper towels to remove excess moisture.

**2.** Combine flour and salt in shallow bowl. Beat eggs in another shallow bowl. Combine panko and cheese in third shallow bowl.

**3.** Coat pickles in flour. Dip in eggs, letting excess drip back into bowl, then coat in panko. Place on prepared baking sheet.

**4.** Bake 15 to 20 minutes or until golden brown. Serve with desired dipping sauce.

**MAKES 4 SERVINGS**

# LETTUCE WRAPS

- **1** tablespoon vegetable oil
- **1** small onion, finely chopped
- **5** ounces cremini mushrooms, finely chopped (about 2 cups)
- **1** pound refrigerated plant-based ground meatless product *or* 1 package (10 ounces) frozen meatless crumbles
- **¼** cup hoisin sauce
- **2** tablespoons soy sauce
- **1** tablespoon rice vinegar
- **1** tablespoon sriracha sauce
- **2** cloves garlic, minced
- **1** teaspoon brown sugar
- **1** teaspoon grated fresh ginger
- **1** teaspoon sesame oil
- **½** cup finely chopped water chestnuts
- **2** green onions, thinly sliced
- **1** head butter lettuce

**1.** Heat oil in large skillet over medium-high heat. Add onion; cook and stir 2 minutes. Add mushrooms; cook about 8 minutes or until lightly browned and liquid has evaporated, stirring occasionally.

**2.** Add meatless product; cook about 8 minutes, stirring to break up into crumbles. Stir in hoisin sauce, soy sauce, vinegar, sriracha, garlic, brown sugar, ginger and sesame oil; cook and stir 4 minutes. Add water chestnuts; cook and stir 2 minutes or until heated through. Remove from heat; stir in green onions.

**3.** Separate lettuce leaves. Spoon about ¼ cup meatless mixture into each lettuce leaf. Serve immediately.

**MAKES 6 TO 8 SERVINGS**

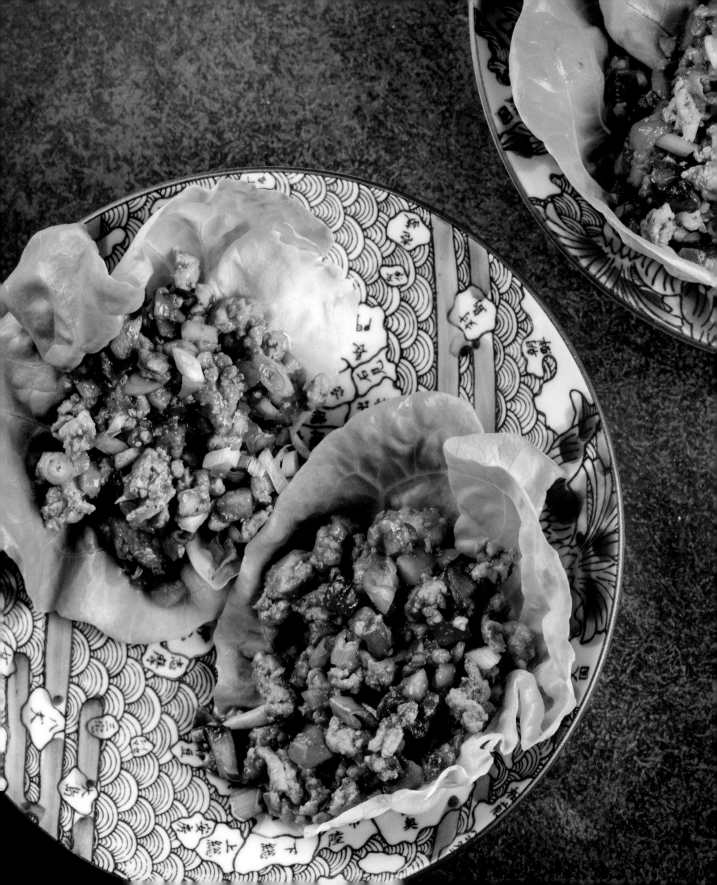

# CREAMY BUFFALO DIP

2 packages (8 ounces each) cream cheese, softened and cut into pieces

1 jar (12 ounces) restaurant-style wing sauce

1 cup ranch dressing

2 packages (8 to 10 ounces each) meatless chicken strips, shredded or finely chopped

2 cups (8 ounces) shredded Cheddar cheese

Tortilla chips

Celery sticks

**1.** Combine cream cheese, wing sauce and ranch dressing in large saucepan; cook over medium-low heat 7 to 10 minutes or until cream cheese is melted and mixture is smooth, whisking frequently.

**2.** Combine meatless chicken and Cheddar cheese in large bowl. Add cream cheese mixture; stir until well blended. Pour into serving bowl; serve warm with tortilla chips and celery sticks.

**MAKES 5 CUPS**

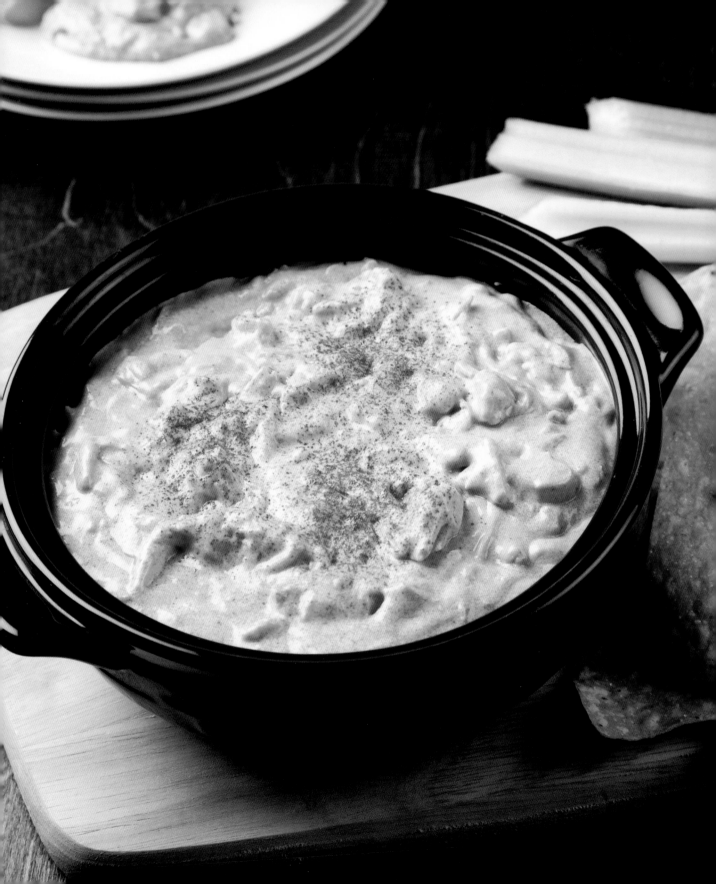

# FRIED CAULIFLOWER WITH GARLIC TAHINI SAUCE

## SAUCE

- ½ **cup tahini**
- ¼ **cup plain Greek yogurt**
- 2 **tablespoons lemon juice**
- 2 **cloves garlic, minced**
- ¼ **teaspoon salt**
- 6 **tablespoons water**
- 1 **tablespoon minced fresh parsley**

## CAULIFLOWER

- 1 **cup all-purpose flour**
- 1½ **teaspoons salt, divided**
  **Pinch black pepper**
- 4 **eggs**
- ¼ **cup water**
- 2 **cups panko bread crumbs**
- 1 **teaspoon ground cumin**
- 1 **teaspoon garlic powder**
- ¼ **teaspoon ground nutmeg**
- 1 **large head cauliflower (2½ pounds), cut into 1-inch florets**
- 1 **quart vegetable oil**

**1.** For sauce, whisk tahini, yogurt, lemon juice, garlic and ¼ teaspoon salt in medium bowl. Whisk in enough water in thin steady stream until sauce is thinned to desired consistency. Stir in parsley.

**2.** For cauliflower, whisk flour, ½ teaspoon salt and pepper in large bowl. Whisk eggs and ¼ cup water in medium bowl. Combine panko, remaining 1 teaspoon salt, cumin, garlic powder and nutmeg in large bowl. Toss cauliflower florets in flour mixture to coat; tap off excess. Dip in egg mixture, letting excess drain back into bowl. Place in panko mixture; toss until coated. Place breaded cauliflower on sheet pan.

**3.** Line another sheet pan with three layers of paper towels. Fill large deep saucepan with 3 inches of oil. Clip deep-fry or candy thermometer to side of pan. Heat over medium-high heat to 350°F; adjust heat to maintain temperature during frying. Add cauliflower in batches; cook 4 minutes, stirring once or twice. Remove with tongs or large slotted spoon; drain on paper towels on prepared sheet pan. Serve warm with sauce.

**MAKES 8 SERVINGS**

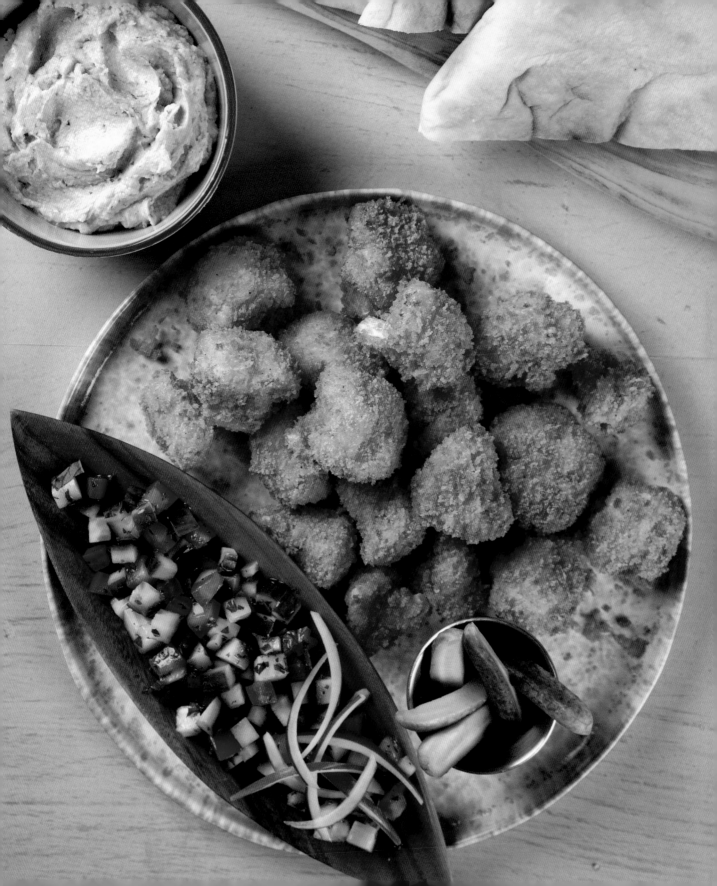

# TEXAS CAVIAR

1 tablespoon vegetable oil

1 cup fresh corn (from 2 to 3 ears)

3 cups cooked black-eyed peas (see Tip)

1 can (15 ounces) black beans

1 cup halved grape tomatoes

1 bell pepper (red, orange, yellow or green), finely chopped

½ cup finely chopped red onion

1 jalapeño pepper, seeded and minced

2 green onions, minced

¼ cup chopped fresh cilantro

2 tablespoons red wine vinegar

1 tablespoon plus 1 teaspoon lime juice, divided

1 teaspoon salt

1 teaspoon sugar

½ teaspoon ground cumin

½ teaspoon dried oregano

2 cloves garlic, minced

¼ cup olive oil

**1.** Heat vegetable oil in large skillet over high heat. Add corn; cook and stir about 3 minutes or until corn is beginning to brown in spots. Place in large bowl. Add beans, tomatoes, bell peppers, red onion, jalapeño, green onions and cilantro.

**2.** Combine vinegar, 1 tablespoon lime juice, 1 teaspoon salt, sugar, cumin, oregano and garlic in small bowl. Whisk in olive oil in thin steady stream until well blended. Pour over vegetables; stir to coat.

**3.** Refrigerate at least 2 hours or overnight. Just before serving, stir in remaining 1 teaspoon lime juice. Taste and season with additional salt, if desired.

**MAKES ABOUT 9 CUPS**

**TIP**

Use 2 (15-ounce) cans, rinsed and drained or cook the beans from dried. Soak 8 ounces of dried beans in salted water at least 4 hours or overnight. Drain beans and place in large saucepan. Cover with water and bring to a boil over high heat. Reduce heat; simmer 45 minutes to 1 hour or until beans are tender. Drain and let cool before using.

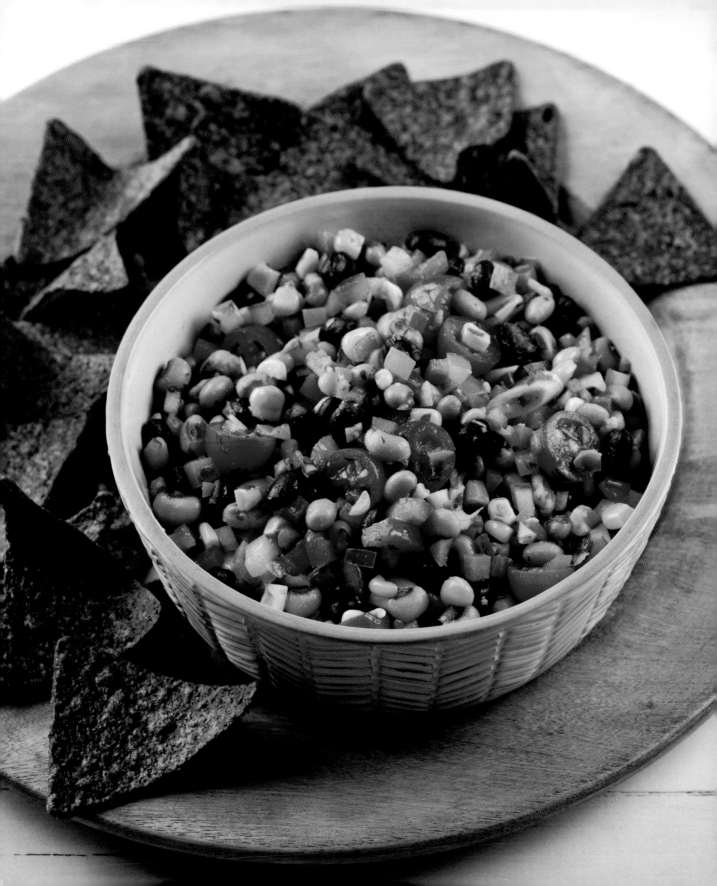

# TEX-MEX NACHOS

1 tablespoon vegetable oil

8 ounces refrigerated plant-based ground meatless product *or* 1 package (10 ounces) frozen meatless crumbles

½ cup chopped onion

2 cloves garlic, minced

2 teaspoons chili powder

1 teaspoon ground cumin

½ teaspoon salt

½ teaspoon dried oregano

1 can (about 15 ounces) kidney beans, rinsed and drained

½ cup corn

½ cup sour cream, divided

2 tablespoons mayonnaise

1 tablespoon lime juice

¼ to ½ teaspoon ground chipotle pepper

½ bag tortilla chips

½ (15-ounce) jar Cheddar cheese dip, warmed

½ cup pico de gallo

¼ cup guacamole

1 cup shredded iceberg lettuce

2 jalapeño peppers, thinly sliced into rings

**1.** Heat oil in large skillet over medium-high heat. Add meatless product, onion and garlic; cook and stir 6 minutes or until onion is tender, breaking up meatless product into crumbles. Add chili powder, cumin, salt and oregano; cook and stir 1 minute. Add beans and corn; reduce heat to medium-low and cook 3 minutes or until heated through.

**2.** For chipotle sauce, combine ¼ cup sour cream, mayonnaise, lime juice and chipotle pepper in small bowl; mix well. Place in small plastic squeeze bottle, if desired.

**3.** Spread tortilla chips on platter or large plate. Top with meatless mixture; drizzle with cheese dip. Top with pico de gallo, guacamole, remaining ¼ cup sour cream, lettuce and jalapeños. Squeeze or dollop chipotle sauce over nachos. Serve immediately.

**MAKES 4 TO 6 SERVINGS**

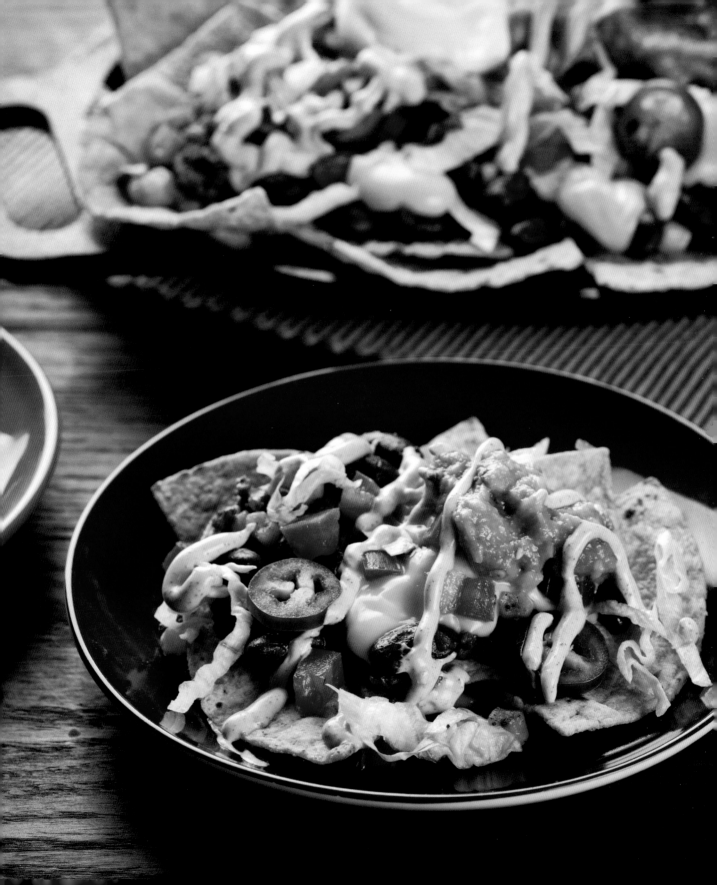

# INDIVIDUAL SPINACH AND BACON QUICHES

1 teaspoon olive oil

½ small onion, diced

1 package (10 ounces) frozen chopped spinach, thawed and squeezed dry

½ teaspoon black pepper

¼ teaspoon salt

⅛ teaspoon ground nutmeg

5 slices vegetarian bacon, cooked according to package directions and chopped

3 eggs

1 container (15 ounces) whole-milk ricotta cheese

2 cups (8 ounces) shredded mozzarella cheese

1 cup grated Parmesan cheese

**1.** Preheat oven to 350°F. Spray 12 standard (2½-inch) muffin cups with nonstick cooking spray.

**2.** Heat oil in large skillet over medium heat. Add onion; cook and stir 5 minutes or until tender. Add spinach, pepper, salt and nutmeg; cook and stir 3 minutes or until liquid is evaporated. Remove from heat. Stir in bacon; set aside to cool.

**3.** Whisk eggs in large bowl. Add cheeses; stir until well blended. Add cooled spinach mixture; mix well. Spoon evenly into prepared muffin cups.

**4.** Bake 40 minutes or until set. Cool in pan 10 minutes. Run thin knife around edges to remove from pan. Serve hot or cold.

**MAKES 12 SERVINGS**

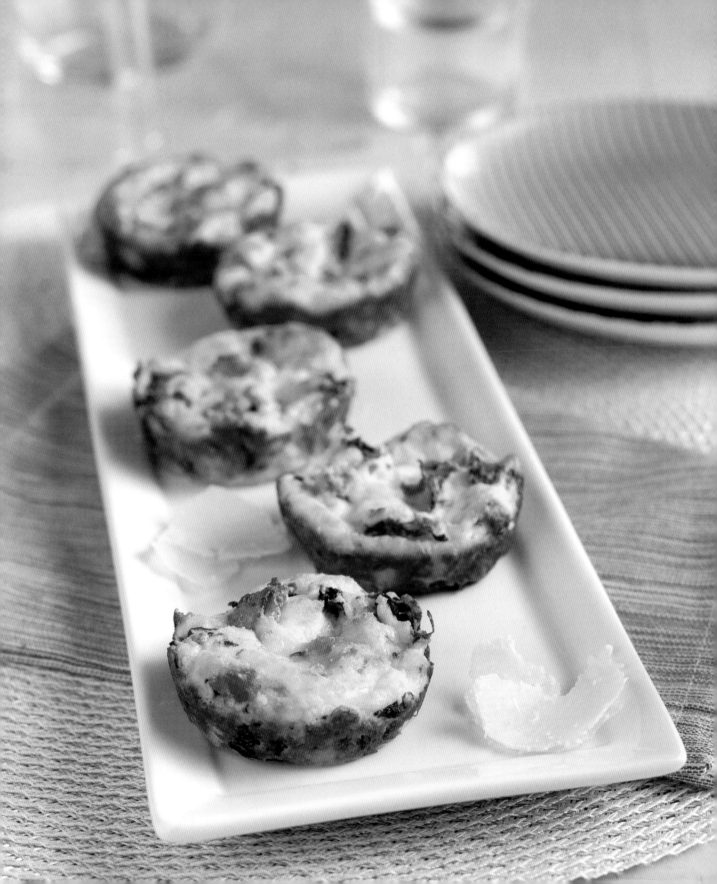

# BUFFALO CAULIFLOWER BITES

¾ cup all-purpose flour

¼ cup cornstarch

1 teaspoon salt

½ teaspoon garlic powder

¼ teaspoon black pepper

1 cup water

1 large head cauliflower (2½ pounds), cut into 1-inch florets

½ cup hot pepper sauce

¼ cup (½ stick) butter, melted

Blue cheese or ranch dressing and celery sticks for serving

**1.** Preheat oven to 450°F. Line sheet pan with foil; spray with nonstick cooking spray.

**2.** Whisk flour, cornstarch, salt, garlic powder and black pepper in large bowl. Whisk in water until smooth and well blended. Add cauliflower to batter in batches; stir to coat. Arrange on prepared sheet pan.

**3.** Bake 20 minutes or until lightly browned. Combine hot pepper sauce and butter in small bowl. Pour over cauliflower; toss until well blended. Bake 5 minutes; stir. Bake 5 minutes more or until cauliflower is glazed and crisp. Serve with blue cheese dressing and celery sticks.

**MAKES 8 SERVINGS**

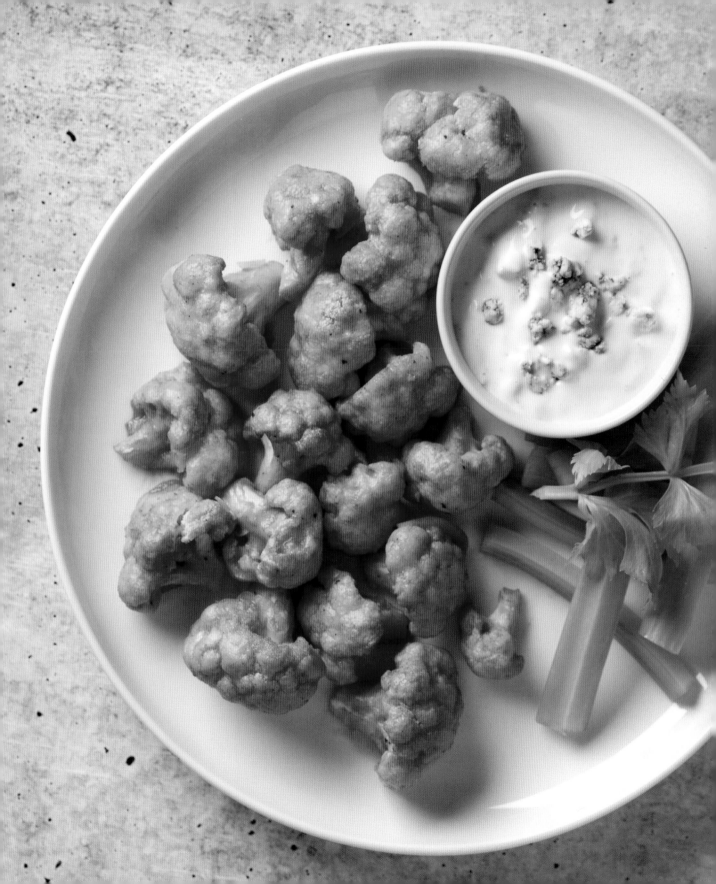

# ARTICHOKE PESTO DIP

3 pieces lavash bread, each about 7×9 inches *or* 4 pita breads

¼ cup plus 2 tablespoons olive oil, divided

¾ teaspoon kosher salt, divided

1 can (14 ounces) artichoke hearts, rinsed and drained

½ cup chopped walnuts, toasted*

¼ cup packed fresh basil leaves

1 clove garlic, minced

2 tablespoons lemon juice

¼ cup grated Parmesan cheese

*To toast walnuts, spread on baking sheet. Bake in preheated 350°F oven 6 to 8 minutes or until golden brown, stirring frequently.

**1.** Preheat oven to 350°F. Line two baking sheets with parchment paper.

**2.** Brush both sides of each piece lavash with 2 tablespoons oil. Sprinkle with ¼ teaspoon salt. Bake 10 minutes or until lavash is crisp and browned, turning and rotating baking sheets after 5 minutes. Cool completely on baking sheets on wire racks.

**3.** Place artichokes, walnuts, basil, garlic, lemon juice and remaining ½ teaspoon salt in food processor; pulse about 12 times until coarsely chopped. With motor running, slowly stream in remaining ¼ cup oil until smooth. Add cheese; pulse until blended.

**4.** Break lavash into chips. Serve with pesto.

**MAKES 6 SERVINGS
(ABOUT 1½ CUPS PESTO)**

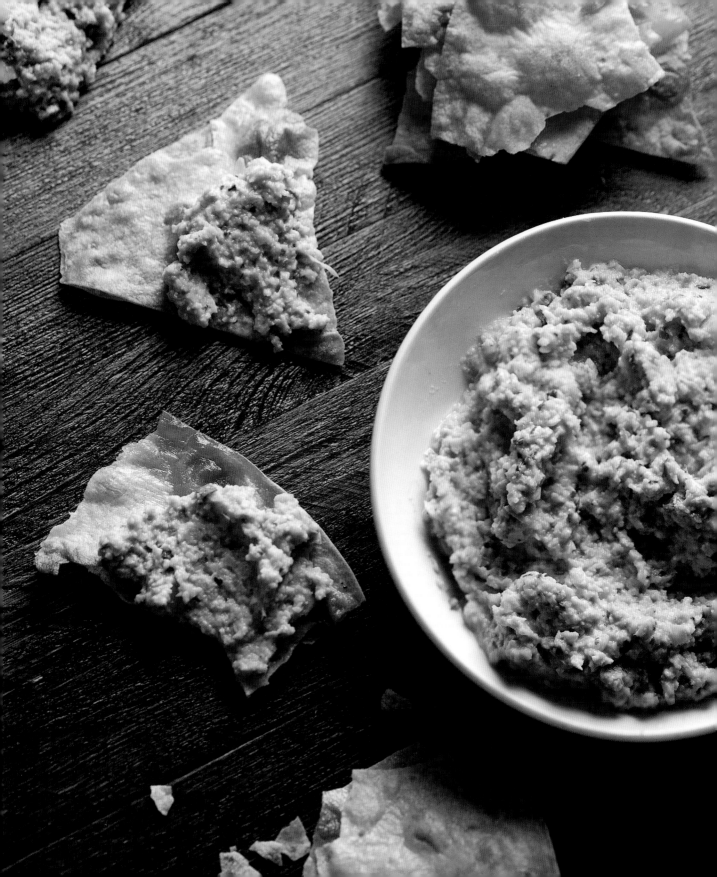

# AVOCADO EGG ROLLS

## DIPPING SAUCE

- ½ **cup cashew nut pieces**
- ½ **cup packed fresh cilantro**
- ¼ **cup honey**
- 2 **green onions, coarsely chopped**
- 2 **cloves garlic**
- 1 **tablespoon white vinegar**
- 1 **teaspoon balsamic vinegar**
- 1 **teaspoon ground cumin**
- ½ **teaspoon tamarind paste**
- ⅛ **teaspoon ground turmeric**
- ¼ **cup olive oil**

## EGG ROLLS

- 2 **avocados, halved and pitted**
- ¼ **cup chopped drained oil-packed sun-dried tomatoes**
- 2 **tablespoons diced red onion**
- 2 **tablespoons chopped fresh cilantro**
- 1 **tablespoon lime juice**
- ¼ **teaspoon salt**
- 10 **egg roll wrappers**
  **Vegetable oil for frying**

**1.** For sauce, combine cashews, cilantro, honey, green onions, garlic, white vinegar, balsamic vinegar, cumin, tamarind paste and turmeric in food processor; process until coarsely chopped. With motor running, drizzle in olive oil in thin steady stream; process until finely chopped and well blended. Refrigerate until ready to use.

**2.** For egg rolls, scoop avocados in medium bowl; coarsely mash with potato masher. Stir in sun-dried tomatoes, red onion, chopped cilantro, lime juice and salt until well blended.

**3.** Working with one at a time, place egg roll wrapper on work surface with one corner facing you. Spread 2 tablespoons filling horizontally across wrapper. Fold short sides over filling and fold up bottom corner over filling. Moisten top edges with water; roll up egg roll, pressing to seal. Refrigerate until ready to cook.

**4.** Heat 2 inches of vegetable oil in large saucepan over medium-high heat to 350°F; adjust heat to maintain temperature. Cook egg rolls in batches about 3 minutes or until golden brown, turning once. Drain on paper towel-lined plate. Cut egg rolls in half diagonally; serve with sauce.

**MAKES 8 TO 10 SERVINGS; 20 PIECES AND 1 CUP SAUCE**

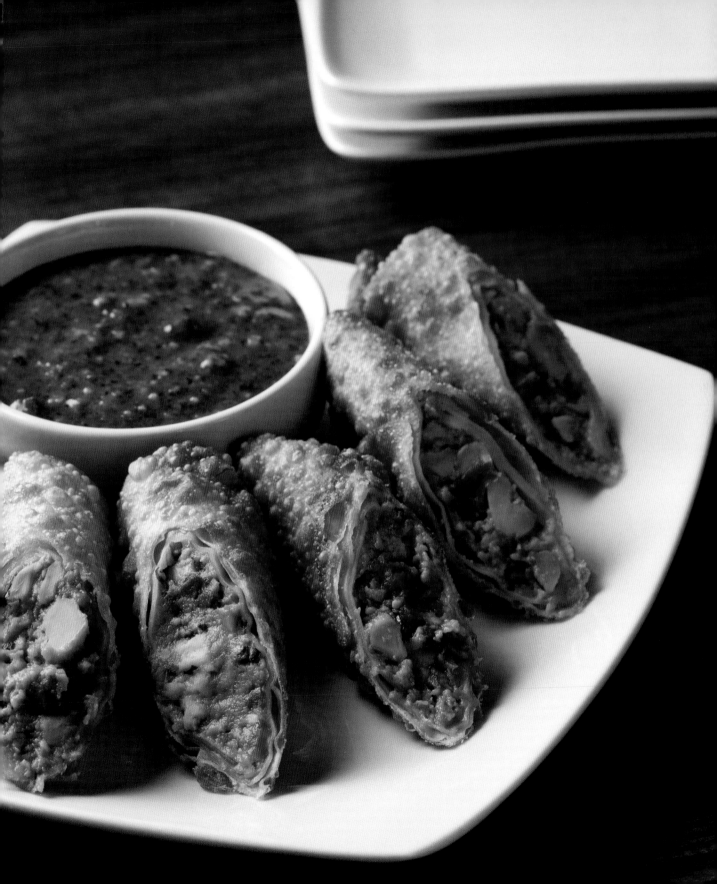

# CAULIFLOWER SOCCA

- **2 cups chickpea flour (besan)**
- **1¾ teaspoons salt**
- **¼ teaspoon black pepper**
- **2 cups water**
- **½ cup olive oil, divided**
- **1½ cups finely chopped cauliflower**
- **1 can (about 15 ounces) chickpeas, rinsed and drained**
- **2 tablespoons chopped fresh cilantro or parsley**

**1.** Whisk chickpea flour, salt and pepper in large bowl to remove any lumps. Whisk in water and ¼ cup oil. Let stand at room temperature at least 30 minutes.

**2.** Meanwhile, preheat oven to 450°F. Place skillet in oven to preheat at least 10 minutes. Pour remaining ¼ cup oil into hot skillet. Add cauliflower and chickpeas. Bake 10 minutes.

**3.** Whisk cilantro into batter; pour batter over cauliflower and chickpeas in skillet. Bake 15 minutes or until edge is lightly browned, top is firm and toothpick inserted into center comes out with moist crumbs. Cut into wedges; serve warm or at room temperature.

**MAKES 8 SERVINGS**

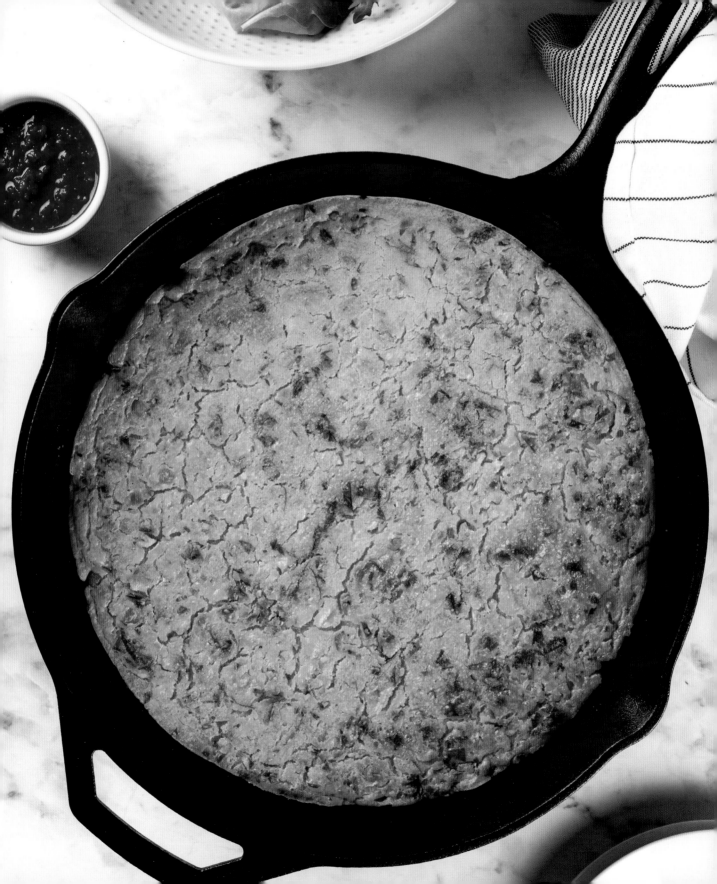

# JALAPEÑO POPPERS

**10** **to 12 fresh jalapeño peppers***

**1** **package (8 ounces) cream cheese, softened**

**1½** **cups (6 ounces) shredded Cheddar cheese, divided**

**2** **green onions, finely chopped**

**½** **teaspoon onion powder**

**¼** **teaspoon salt**

**⅛** **teaspoon garlic powder**

**6** **slices vegetarian bacon, cooked according to package directions and finely chopped**

**2** **tablespoons plain dry bread crumbs (optional)**

**2** **tablespoons grated Parmesan or Romano cheese**

**\*For large jalapeño peppers, use 10. For small peppers, use 12.**

**1.** Preheat oven to 375°F. Line baking sheet with parchment paper or foil.

**2.** Cut each jalapeño in half lengthwise; remove ribs and seeds.

**3.** Combine cream cheese, 1 cup Cheddar cheese, green onions, onion powder, salt and garlic powder in medium bowl. Stir in bacon. Fill each jalapeño half with about 1 tablespoon cheese mixture. Place on prepared baking sheet. Sprinkle with remaining ½ cup Cheddar cheese, bread crumbs, if desired, and Parmesan cheese.

**4.** Bake 10 to 12 minutes or until cheese is melted but jalapeños are still firm.

**MAKES 20 TO 24 POPPERS**

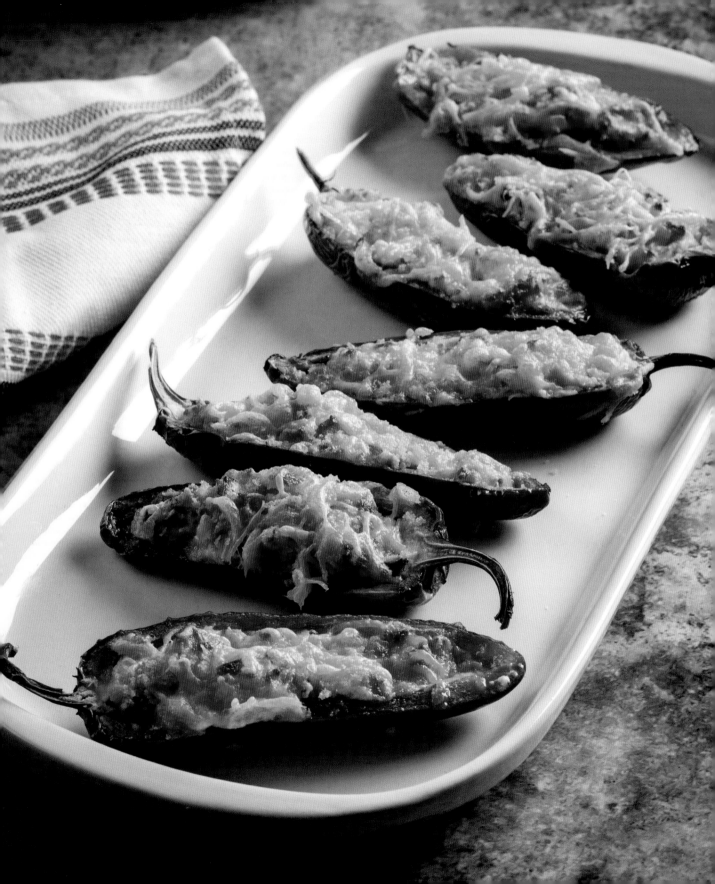

# METRIC CONVERSION CHART

## VOLUME MEASUREMENTS (dry)

$\frac{1}{8}$ teaspoon = 0.5 mL
$\frac{1}{4}$ teaspoon = 1 mL
$\frac{1}{2}$ teaspoon = 2 mL
$\frac{3}{4}$ teaspoon = 4 mL
1 teaspoon = 5 mL
1 tablespoon = 15 mL
2 tablespoons = 30 mL
$\frac{1}{4}$ cup = 60 mL
$\frac{1}{3}$ cup = 75 mL
$\frac{1}{2}$ cup = 125 mL
$\frac{2}{3}$ cup = 150 mL
$\frac{3}{4}$ cup = 175 mL
1 cup = 250 mL
2 cups = 1 pint = 500 mL
3 cups = 750 mL
4 cups = 1 quart = 1 L

## VOLUME MEASUREMENTS (fluid)

1 fluid ounce (2 tablespoons) = 30 mL
4 fluid ounces ($\frac{1}{2}$ cup) = 125 mL
8 fluid ounces (1 cup) = 250 mL
12 fluid ounces ($1\frac{1}{2}$ cups) = 375 mL
16 fluid ounces (2 cups) = 500 mL

## WEIGHTS (mass)

$\frac{1}{2}$ ounce = 15 g
1 ounce = 30 g
3 ounces = 90 g
4 ounces = 120 g
8 ounces = 225 g
10 ounces = 285 g
12 ounces = 360 g
16 ounces = 1 pound = 450 g

## DIMENSIONS

$\frac{1}{16}$ inch = 2 mm
$\frac{1}{8}$ inch = 3 mm
$\frac{1}{4}$ inch = 6 mm
$\frac{1}{2}$ inch = 1.5 cm
$\frac{3}{4}$ inch = 2 cm
1 inch = 2.5 cm

## OVEN TEMPERATURES

250°F = 120°C
275°F = 140°C
300°F = 150°C
325°F = 160°C
350°F = 180°C
375°F = 190°C
400°F = 200°C
425°F = 220°C
450°F = 230°C

## BAKING PAN SIZES

| Utensil | Size in Inches/Quarts | Metric Volume | Size in Centimeters |
|---|---|---|---|
| Baking or Cake Pan (square or rectangular) | 8×8×2 | 2 L | 20×20×5 |
| | 9×9×2 | 2.5 L | 23×23×5 |
| | 12×8×2 | 3 L | 30×20×5 |
| | 13×9×2 | 3.5 L | 33×23×5 |
| Loaf Pan | 8×4×3 | 1.5 L | 20×10×7 |
| | 9×5×3 | 2 L | 23×13×7 |
| Round Layer Cake Pan | 8×1½ | 1.2 L | 20×4 |
| | 9×1½ | 1.5 L | 23×4 |
| Pie Plate | 8×1¼ | 750 mL | 20×3 |
| | 9×1¼ | 1 L | 23×3 |
| Baking Dish or Casserole | 1 quart | 1 L | — |
| | 1½ quart | 1.5 L | — |
| | 2 quart | 2 L | — |